ORL

OXFORD RHEUMATOLOGY LIBRARY

Rheumatoid Arthritis

Oxford University Press makes no representation, express or implied, that the drug dosages in this book are correct. Readers must therefore always check the product information and clinical procedures with the most up-to-date published product information and data sheets provided by the manufacturers and the most recent codes of conduct and safety regulations. The authors and the publishers do not accept responsibility or legal liability for any errors in the text or for the misuse or misapplication of material in this work.

▶ Except where otherwise stated, drug doses and recommendations are for the non-pregnant adult who is not breastfeeding.

▶ Occasionally in our clinical practice we may use drugs at dosages outside of their licensed or BNF dosage ranges. In these cases we follow local agreed clinical protocols. However, we suggest that you always need the Summary of Product Characteristics and British National Formulary monographs before using any drug with which you are unfamiliar.

O R L

OXFORD RHEUMATOLOGY LIBRARY

Rheumatoid Arthritis

Edited by

Raashid Luqmani

Consultant Rheumatologist and Senior Lecturer,
Rheumatology Department,
Nuffield Orthopaedic Centre,
Oxford, UK

Theodore Pincus

Clinical Professor of Medicine,
Director of Outcomes Research,
Division of Rheumatology New York University,
Hospital for Joint Diseases, New York, USA

Maarten Boers

Professor of Clinical Epidemiology,
Department of Clinical Epidemiology
and Biostatistics, VU University Medical Center
Amsterdam, the Netherlands

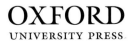

OXFORD
UNIVERSITY PRESS

OXFORD
UNIVERSITY PRESS

Great Clarendon Street, Oxford OX2 6DP

Oxford University Press is a department of the University of Oxford.
It furthers the University's objective of excellence in research, scholarship,
and education by publishing worldwide in

Oxford New York

Auckland Cape Town Dar es Salaam Hong Kong Karachi
Kuala Lumpur Madrid Melbourne Mexico City Nairobi
New Delhi Shanghai Taipei Toronto

With offices in

Argentina Austria Brazil Chile Czech Republic France Greece
Guatemala Hungary Italy Japan Poland Portugal Singapore
South Korea Switzerland Thailand Turkey Ukraine Vietnam

Oxford is a registered trade mark of Oxford University Press
in the UK and in certain other countries

Published in the United States
by Oxford University Press Inc., New York

British Library Cataloguing in Publication Data

Data available

Library of Congress Cataloging in Publication Data

Data available

Typeset by Newgen Imaging Systems (P) Ltd., Chennai, India
Printed in Great Britain
on acid-free paper by
Ashford Colour Press Ltd, Gosport, Hampshire

ISBN 978–0–19–955675–5

10 9 8 7 6 5 4 3 2

Whilst every effort has been made to ensure that the contents of this book are as
complete, accurate and-up-to-date as possible at the date of writing. Oxford
University Press is not able to give any guarantee or assurance that such is the case.
Readers are urged to take appropriately qualified medical advice in all cases. The
information in this book is intended to be useful to the general reader, but should
not be used as a means of self-diagnosis or for the prescription of medication.

Contents

Preface

A short pocketbook on rheumatoid arthritis (RA) is of practical value to many health care practitioners. RA is a common rheumatic disease affecting around 0.5% of total polulation; 1–2% of the adult population and resulting in significant disability in the absence of adequate therapy. Recent advances in our understanding of the pathogenesis of RA mean that therapeutic agents are now being used to target specific disease mechanisms, and new agents are being designed based on greater understanding of the underlying pathogenesis of the disease. Increasing use of intensive conventional therapy and the advent of more advanced biologic agents has altered our expectation of the drug treatment of RA. In line with improvements in drug therapy, the multidisciplinary team approach including physiotherapy, occupational therapy and nurse specialist can be important to patient management. The book provides a summary of our current understanding of the pathogenesis of the disease, including advances in the genetics of RA; disease mechanisms; clinical features for diagnosis and assessment, followed by the role of laboratory investigations and imaging; a therapy-based section covering pain management, use of anti inflammatory drugs, role of disease modifying anti-rheumatic drugs (DMARDs), glucocorticoids and biologic agents; multidisciplinary care; and the long term monitoring of drug toxicity and screening of patients for relevant co-morbidities. Prognosis and long term effects on ability to work and live a normal life are discussed.

The general approach is similar to other books in this series with short notes, summary tables with key points, and illustrations showing important mechanisms of disease.

The book is suitable for primary care physicians, trainees in rheumatology and in orthopaedics, specialist practitioners and therapists involved in the care of patients with RA.

Acknowledgements

We are indebted to our families for ongoing support.

We acknowledge the considerable assistance from Mr Paul Cooper, Medical Illustration department, Nuffield Orthopaedic Centre, Oxford.

We acknowledge the help of Gill Rowbotham for providing expert advice on chapter 7.

We acknowledge Peter Stevenson of OUP for support and encouragement.

We are grateful to Dr Rachel Benamore for supplying some of the chest X-rays and CT scans.

Contributors

Professor Maarten Boers,
Professor of Clinical
Epidemiology,
VU University Medical Centre,
Amsterdam, Netherlands

Professor Matthew Brown,
Professor of Immunogenetics,
University of Queensland,
Brisbane, Australia

Mr Tom Cadoux-Hudson,
Consultant Neruosurgeon,
Oxford Radcliffe Hospital,
Oxford, UK

Ms Jane Flynn,
Specialist Practitioner
in Rheumatology,
Nuffield Orthopaedic Centre,
Oxford, UK

Dr Nicola Goodson,
Senior Lecturer in Rheumatology
and Honorary Consultant
Rheumatologist,
University Hospital Aintree,
Liverpool, UK

Mr Roger Gundle,
Consultant Orthopaedic Surgeon,
Nuffield Orthopaedic Centre,
Oxford, UK

Mrs Sheena Hennell,
Rheumatology Specialist Nurse,
Royal Liverpool
University Hospital,
Liverpool, UK

Dr Gabrielle Kingsley,
Reader in Rheumatology Medicine,
Kings College London, UK

Mr Chris Little,
Consultant Orthopaedic Surgeon,
Nuffield Orthopaedic Centre,
Oxford, UK

Dr Raashid Luqmani,
Consultant Rheumatologist
and Senior Lecturer in
Rheumatology,
Nuffield Orthopaedic Centre,
Oxford, UK

Mr Ian McNab,
Consultant Orthopaedic Surgeon,
Nuffield Orthopaedic Centre,
Oxford, UK

Mr Hemant Pandit,
Research Fellow in Orthopaedics,
Nuffield Orthopaedic Centre,
Oxford, UK

Professor Theodore Pincus,
Clinical Professor of Medicine,
Division of Rheumatology,
New York University,
Hospital for Joint Diseases,
New York, USA

Professor David L Scott,
Professor of Rheumatology,
Kings College London, UK

Mr Bob Sharp,
Consultant Orthopaedic Surgeon,
Nuffield Orthopaedic Centre,
Oxford, UK

CONTRIBUTORS

Ms Zoe Stableford,
Podiatrist,
Salford Royal Hospitals
NHS Trust, UK

Dr Catherine Swales,
Lecturer in Rheumatology,
Nuffield Orthopaedic Centre,
Oxford, UK

Professor Paul P Tak,
Professor of Medicine,
Division of Clinical Immunology
and Rheumatology Academic
Medical Center,
University of Amsterdam,
Amsterdam, Netherlands

Professor Peter Taylor,
Professor in Experimental
Rheumatology,
Kennedy Institute
of Rheumatology,
London, UK

Professor Paul Wordsworth,
Professor of Rheumatology,
University of Oxford,
Oxford, UK

Abbreviations

ACPA	Anti-citrullinated protein/peptide antibody
ACR	American College of Rheumatology
ADL	Activities of daily living
ARA	American Rheumatism Association
CDAI	Clinical disease activity index
CIA	Collagen-induced arthritis
COX	Cyclo-oxygenase
CRP	C-reactive protein
CVD	Cardiovascular disease
DALY	Disability Adjusted Life Years
DAS28	Disease activity score using 28 joint counts
DMARDs	Disease-modifying anti-rheumatic drugs
ESR	Erythrocyte sedimentation rate
HAD	Hospital Anxiety and Depression Scale
HAQ	Health Assessment Questionnaire
HAQ-DI	HAQ disability index
HRCT	High Resolution Computerised Tomography
LFN	leflunomide
MDHAQ	Multidimensional HAQ
MTX	methotrexate
NRAS	National Rheumatoid Arthritis Society
NSAIDs	Non-steroidal anti-inflammatory drugs
NSIP	Non specific interstitial pneumonia
QALY	Quality Adjusted Life Years
RA	Rheumatoid arthritis
SSZ	Sulfasalazine
TB	Tuberculosis
TENS	Trans cutaneous electrical nerve stimulation
UIP	Usual interstitial pneumonia

Chapter 1

Epidemiology, genetics and economic burden of rheumatoid arthritis

Matthew Brown and Maarten Boers

1

Key points

- Rheumatoid arthritis occurs in 1–2% of the population worldwide
- The average age of incident cases is 50–55 years but may be rising
- RA is more common in women than men, and in men is somewhat more common in cigarette smokers
- The economic burden of RA is enormous and work disability is common
- The natural history of RA includes a risk of premature mortality (by 5–10 years)
- The most significant recognized predictor of premature mortality and work disability is functional disability
- 60% of the risk of developing RA appears to be due to genetic factors
- Genes involved in disease susceptibility include HLA-DRB1, with a strong link to the presence of anti-cyclic citrullinated peptide antibodies (ACPA)
- Most patients have positive tests for rheumatoid factor and ACPA, but more than 30% are negative.

1.1 Incidence and prevalence

The prevalence of rheumatoid arthritis (RA) is reported to be 0.5–1.0% in most populations worldwide. North American data from Rochester, Minnesota, suggests that rheumatoid arthritis is found in 0.85% of adults in that population and that >2 million Americans have the disease. In the United Kingdom a similar prevalence (0.8%) has been reported, and it is thought that 475,000 people have the disease. Several studies have suggested that the prevalence of rheumatoid arthritis is falling. The prevalence in Rochester, Minnesota in 1985 was 1.07%, approximately 20% higher than 10 years later. This reduction has also been observed in other countries including England and Finland. The reduction in RA prevalence appears to be greatest in women, with little reduction in the prevalence in men. In public health terms, RA results in an enormous burden of disability, particularly work disability.

Whilst RA occurs in all races world-wide, there are significant differences in its prevalence in different populations. It is not known if this is due to genetic differences between populations, or environmental differences in the countries concerned, or possibly due to ascertainment bias. RA appears to be less common in Asia and Southern Europe than in America and Northern Europe. In China the prevalence is 0.28%, India 0.5%, and in the Philippines only 0.17%. In rural Africans and Australian Aboriginals the disease is reported to be uncommon, whilst it is more common in African Americans. Recent genetic data suggests that increased European genetic admixture may be responsible for the higher prevalence of RA in African Americans than Africans themselves.

The average age of cases of prevalent RA is 66.8 years in North America, over 5 years older than it had been in 1985. The incidence of RA increases throughout life, with a peak at about age 50–55 years and thus the increase in age of prevalent cases may in part be due to the increasing age of the whole population. Studies from the Norfolk Arthritis Registry in England indicate that the annual incidence in women is 36/100,000, and in men 14/100,000. Data from this registry indicate that the incidence in women peaks at 65–74 years of age, that the annual incidence in men is very low under 45 years of age (≤3/100,000), and that over the age of 75 years, the incidence is higher in men than women. There is also a suggestion of a temporal trend for rheumatoid arthritis to become less severe, with lower prevalence of rheumatoid nodules, seropositivity, elevated erythocyte sedimentation rate and rheumatoid vasculitis observed. These trends were seen even before the widespread advances in treatments.

RA is more common in women. Prior to the menopause, the gender ratio is about 4:1, which declines in postmenopausal years to about 2:1. There is an association between cigarette smoking and the risk of RA in men, but this association is weaker in women if present at all. Mortality in RA is increased in both men and women, with the most common cause of death being cardiovascular disease, even in early disease. The likelihood of cardiovascular disease as a cause of death is 40–50%, similar to the general population, except that it occurs 4–10 years earlier compared with the general population. Women develop more disability, and men are thought more likely to enter remission.

1.2 Economic burden of RA

The mean annual per patient cost of RA in developed countries ranges between 15,000–25,000 Euros (2006 estimates). The cost varies widely between countries depending on the health care system, availability of high cost biologic agents, labour costs and informal care costs (costs of unpaid care). The average cost in the United Kingdom is estimated at 16,500 Euros per annum, and in the United States, 21,000 Euros per annum. The average cost in western European countries is much higher than in Eastern Europe (17,000 Euros vs. 5,000 Euros per annum). On average in European countries, drug costs constitute 14% of the total, other medical costs 21%, informal care costs 19%, indirect costs 32% (e.g. reduced employment) and non-medical care costs 14%. The greater cost in the United States is as a result of higher medication costs, due to greater use of biological agents, as well as the administrative costs. Given the high prevalence of RA, the overall cost of the disease is substantial. The total health care cost was estimated to be 45 billion Euros in Europe and 42 billion Euros in the United States in 2006.

RA severely impacts on quality of life amongst those affected. This can be measured using the 'Quality Adjusted Life Years' (QALY) or 'Disability Adjusted Life Years' (DALY), which are terms with no meaning to individuals but which assist in comparing impact on quality of life in different diseases. World Health Organization estimates suggest that RA is responsible for 0.8% of DALY's lost per annum and 0.1% of mortality in European countries. In terms of QALY's, RA is associated with similar loss of QALY's per individual to multiple sclerosis and chronic ischaemic heart disease, and is amongst the most severe diseases in terms of reduction in quality of life.

Patients with RA have a high rate of work disability, but there is some evidence that this trend can be prevented by successful treatment of early arthritis. Five years after disease onset, 20% of patients have given up their jobs. The risk of unemployment is 25% greater in RA, compared to controls, and more patients with RA work only part-time. Many patients (in some series up to 50%) of those patients who stop working do so within the first 5 years of disease, emphasizing the need for early assistance and interventions to help people remain within the workforce. Work disability is related more to occupation, age, disease status, and the social system than to disease activity or gender (see chapter 7). In a study of disability as measured using the Health Assessment Questionnaire (HAQ), worse HAQ scores were associated with more work disability in Finland, compared to the United States, where awarding of work disability payments is less likely.

Recently, the concept of 'presenteeism' has been introduced. It describes the phenomenon of employees who are at work but performing poorly due to their disease. This may be an important and as yet unmeasured contributor to societal cost of the disease.

RA has many effects on the family, including the greater demands placed on families in care provision, reduced income, and the impact of the disease on the patient's psychosocial function. There does not appear to be an increase in family dysfunction. Divorce rates in RA may be only slightly higher than in the general population, but patients with RA who do divorce are much less likely to remarry compared to unaffected individuals.

1.3 Genetic factors in RA

RA is known to run strongly in families, and to be highly heritable. Familiality can be measured using the sibling recurrence risk ratio, λS, which is the recurrence rate in siblings of cases, compared with the population frequency of the disease, and for RA, that risk is 14. Recurrence risk estimates for relatives of cases are shown in Table 1.1.

Familiality is caused by shared genes and environmental factors. The magnitude of the genetic component is measured as 'heritability', which in RA is about 60% (i.e. 60% of the risk of developing RA appears to be due to genetic factors).

Several genes are known to be associated with the development of RA (see Box 1.1).

Those with the biggest contributions are HLA-DRB1 and PTPN22, which will be discussed in more detail.

1.3.1 HLA-DRB1

The major histocompatibility complex (MHC) is situated on chromosome 6 (6p21.3) and extends over 3.6Mb (see Figure 1.1). It is a highly gene dense region containing about 224 genes, 40% of which are predicted to have immunoregulatory functions. Approximately 30% of the genetic risk for RA appears to be encoded within the MHC.

Following the first reports that RA is associated with the broad HLA-DR specificity Dw4, higher resolution genetic typing of HLA-DRB1 demonstrated that different HLA-DR4 variants are not equally associated with RA, and that some non-DR4 HLA-DRB1 alleles are also associated with disease. Gregersen and colleagues first proposed

Table 1.1 Approximate risk estimates for development of RA in relatives of a patient with established RA	
Identical twin	30%
Sibling	4%
Parent/child	4.7%
Second degree relatives	1.9%
Third degree relatives	1.07%

> **Box 1.1 Genes associated with the development and severity of RA**
>
> - HLA-DRB1
> - PTPN22
> - PADI4
> - CCL21
> - CDK6
> - CD40
> - C-REL
> - CTLA4
> - IL12RB
> - MMEL1/TNFRS14
> - PRKCQ
> - STAT4
> - TNFAIP3/OLIG3
> - TRAF1-C5
> - 4Q27 (IL2/21)
> - 12Q13 (KIF5A, PIP4K2C)

the unifying 'shared epitope' (SE) hypothesis, demonstrating that RA is associated with specific HLA-DRB1 (DRB1) alleles that encode a conserved sequence of amino acids termed the SE, (^{70}QRRAA^{74}, ^{70}RRRAA^{74} or ^{70}QKRAA^{74}) which comprise residues 70-74 in the third hypervariable region (HVR3) of the DRβ1 chain. The alleles carrying this nucleotide sequence are DRB1*0401, *0404, *0405, *0408, *0101, *0102, *1402, *09 and *1001.

This hypothesis does not fully explain characteristics of the MHC associations of RA. In particular, it does not explain the differential strength of association of SE-carrying DRB1 alleles. Carriage of DRB1*0401/DRX, where X is a non-SE encoding allele, has a relative risk (RR) for developing RA of 4.7. For DRB1*0404/DRX the RR=5.0, *0401/*0401 the RR=18.8, for DRB1*0401/DRB1*0404 heterozygotes the RR=31, and for *0404,5,8/*0404,5,8 the RR=36.2. It also has been suggested that heterozygosity for particular SE-carrying alleles (particularly *0401/*0404) carries a greater risk than homozygosity for the individual alleles alone. The combinations *0401/*0401, *0401/*0404, and *0101/*0401 are particularly associated with increased risk of rheumatoid vasculitis (odds ratio ~4). The absolute risk of developing RA if carrying a SE encoding allele is 1 in 20 for *0404, 1 in 35 for *0401, and 1 in 80 for *0101.

It is likely that further MHC genes are involved in RA-susceptibility, and that either they interact differently with, or are carried on different haplotypes by, different SE-carrying alleles. No explanation has yet been proven for this association, but it is most likely that the SE-carrying alleles are predisposed to presenting particular arthritogenic peptides.

Figure 1.1 The major histocompatibility complex (MHC) is situated on chromosome 6 (6p21.3) and extends over 3.6Mb

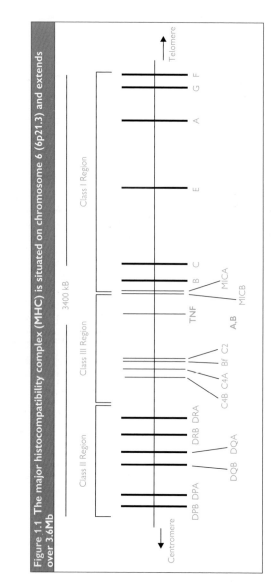

Recently it has been demonstrated that the HLA-DRB1 association with RA is restricted to cases which are ACPA positive, and that in this group there is an interaction between cigarette smoking, shared-epitope status, and the development of RA. Smoking increases the risk of RA, especially in particular genetically-defined groups. Shared-epitope carriers who smoke are more likely to develop ACPA and bone erosions than non-smokers. Both shared-epitope status and ACPA carriage are associated with increased rates of erosive RA. ACPA positive RA has thus been identified as a genetically distinct subset of RA. This group also has increased mortality in RA, particularly from coronary vascular disease (hazards ratio 7.8x), and thus reflect a group that should probably be targeted for vascular disease preventative interventions (see Chapter 8 on comorbidity).

1.3.2 Protein Tyrosine Phosphatase 22 (*PTPN22*)

The gene *PTPN22* was found to be associated with RA having originally been identified as a susceptibility gene for type 1 diabetes mellitus. It encodes a 110-kD cytoplasmic protein tyrosine phosphatase (Lyp) that is thought to function as a down-regulator of T-cell receptor dependent responses through interaction with a negative regulatory kinase, Csk. The associated allele is found in 17% of healthy white individuals compared with 28% of RA cases, so there is increased risk, although 5 out of 7 RA cases don't carry the disease-associated genetic variant. This gene is also associated with a variety of other autoimmune diseases including systemic lupus erythematosus, Addison's disease and Hashimoto's thyroiditis, in addition to RA and type 1 diabetes mellitus, helping to explain the tendency for these conditions to segregate together.

There is strong evidence of interaction between *PTPN22* and shared-epitope in the development of RA, with carriers of risk alleles at both loci being at more than 20-times greater risk of having ACPA positive RA than non-carriers, with carriers of alleles at either locus alone having intermediate risk. Cigarette smoke may also interact with *PTPN22*, influencing the risk of developing ACPA positive RA, but this is not fully established.

Studying populations with different genetic architecture is a widely used strategy to help clarify disease-associations, including pinpointing specific regions of genes involved in disease-risk, and through identification of genes whose polymorphism may be population-restricted. Studies of HLA-DRB1 allelic associations with RA in different ethnic groups have been particularly helpful in determining the likely mechanism explaining the association of this gene with RA, leading to the formulation of the 'shared-epitope' hypothesis. The gene *PADI4* has been comprehensively demonstrated to be associated with RA in Japanese and Korean populations, but not in Caucasians. The enzyme

PADI4 citrullinates peptides, antibodies against which (ACPA) are highly specific for RA. The discovery of the association of *PADI4* with RA has been interpreted to suggest that ACPA are important in disease pathogenesis, and not merely an immunological epiphenomenon. A further example of interethnic differences in the genetic determinants of RA-susceptibility involves the gene *PTPN22*, which clearly is a major gene influencing RA risk in Caucasians but is not associated with RA in Japanese. This appears to be because the major associated SNP in *PTPN22* is not polymorphic in Japanese. The absence of this genetic effect raises the possibility that studies in Asian populations may be particularly informative of novel genetic variants involved in RA.

A rapidly increasing number of genes are now known to be involved in the development of RA and in determining its radiographic severity (see Box 1.1). A region of chromosome 6q has recently been demonstrated to harbour an RA-susceptibility gene, thought to be *TNFAIP3*. It is likely that more than one gene is encoded in this region which is associated with RA, complicating the identification of the principal variants. There is also strong evidence that further genes within the MHC in addition to *DRB1* are associated with RA. Research in this area is complicated by the strong and varied linkage disequilibrium across the MHC associated with different *DRB1* shared epitope alleles.

It is clear that many other genes remain to be identified, probably contributing small individual effects, but collectively increasing the population risk of RA. There is also considerable interest in genetic determinants of disease severity. *DRB1* is associated with radiographic severity (but not with functional diability), though whether that risk is independent of the association with ACPA remains unclear. A further area of research interest is in pharmacogenetics, particularly with regard to TNF-blockade response. Thus far only candidate gene studies have been performed, and no convincing evidence has been demonstrated to implicate any particular gene.

1.4 Environmental factors and RA

The substantial non-heritable fraction of the risk of developing RA indicates that there must be major environmental factors involved in the disease onset. Unlike genetics, which is a finite (if massive) area of research, there are no obvious limits as to the type or mechanism underlying environmental factors potentially involved in RA susceptibility. There are several infectious conditions (typically self limiting viral arthropathies such as parvovirus and chronic hepatitis B infection) that mimic RA, suggesting a potential viral aetiology for RA itself. However 'outbreaks' of RA are so few as to be likely to be chance clusters, and the worldwide distribution of the disease suggests that the environmental agents involved must be ubiquitous.

The only established environmental agent involved in RA is smoking. Cigarette smoking, particularly amongst males that carry shared-epitope alleles, is a risk factor for RA. Given that the peptides against which ACPA are targeted are thought to develop mainly against fibrinogen formed in the synovium, the hypothesis has been raised that cigarette smoking increases RA risk by increasing intravascular fibrinogen formation. There is also evidence that it upregulates PADI enzymes, which convert arginine to citrulline in peptides and proteins such as fibrinogen, against which ACPA are directed.

Because smoking influences only the risk of seropositive RA, and most patients with RA have not previously smoked, it is evident that other environmental triggers must also be involved. At this stage we have few clues as to what they are.

Further reading

Begovich AB, Carlton VE, Honigberg LA, et al. A mis-sense single-nucleotide polymorphism in a gene encoding a protein tyrosine phosphatase (PTPN22) is associated with rheumatoid arthritis. Am J Hum Genet 2004; 75(2): 330–7.

Harrison B, Symmons D. Early inflammatory polyarthritis: results from the Norfolk Arthritis Register with a review of the literature. II. Outcome at three years. Rheumatology (Oxford) 2000; 39(9): 939–49.

Helmick CG, Felson DT, Lawrence RC, et al. Estimates of the prevalence of arthritis and other rheumatic conditions in the United States. Part I. Arthritis Rheum 2008; 58(1): 15–25.

Klareskog L, Stolt P, Lundberg K, et al. A new model for an etiology of rheumatoid arthritis: smoking may trigger HLA-DR (shared epitope)-restricted immune reactions to autoantigens modified by citrullination. Arthritis Rheum 2006; 54(1): 38–46.

Nishimura K, Sugiyama D, Kogata Y, Tsuji G, Nakazawa T, Kawano S et al. Meta-analysis: Diagnostic accuracy of anti-cyclic citrullinated peptide antibody and rheumatoid factor for rheumatoid arthritis. Ann Intern Med 2007; 146(11): 797–808.

Silman AJ. Forty-six million Americans have arthritis: true or false? Arthritis Rheum 2008; 58(5): 1220–5.

Symmons D, Harrison B. Early inflammatory polyarthritis: results from the Norfolk arthritis register with a review of the literature. I. Risk factors for the development of inflammatory polyarthritis and rheumatoid arthritis. Rheumatology (Oxford) 2000; 39(8): 835–43.

Chapter 2

The pathogenesis of rheumatoid arthritis

Catherine Swales, Paul Wordsworth
and Raashid Luqmani

Key points

- Many cell types and mediators are implicated in the pathogenesis of rheumatoid arthritis
- Tumour necrosis factor alpha (TNFα) is currently identified as one the most important cytokines responsible for mediating inflammation and damage in arthritis
- Interleukin-17 (IL-17) has been found to regulate many cytokines including TNFα
- T helper 17 (T_H17) and T helper 1 (T_H1) cells are the dominant T cell subsets in rheumatoid synovium
- Novel mechanisms for perpetuation of arthritis are being elucidated, which may lead to more effective therapeutic strategies in future.

Rheumatoid arthritis (RA) is a classic autoimmune disease, with abnormalities of both the cellular and humoral components of immunity.

Cellular immunity relies on the thymus to delete self-reactive lymphocytes, forming (thymus-dependent) T cells. T cells are responsible either for direct destruction of infected cells (cytotoxic or T_C cells) or orchestration of further immune responses through cytokine release (helper or T_H cells). Cytokines such as tumour necrosis factor alpha (TNFα) and the interleukins (ILs) are soluble mediators that act as stimulatory or inhibitory signals between cells; when they affect chemotaxis they are referred to as chemokines. Regulatory T cells induce tolerance to antigens by reducing the effects of fully functional effector T cells. In this way, they are important in the maintenance of peripheral tolerance and prevention of autoimmunity.

Humoral immunity relies on cellular maturation in the bone marrow, resulting in (bone marrow-dependent) B cells. Although the primary role of B cells is antibody formation, they also contribute to inflammation by cytokine release, antigen presentation and modulation of T cells.

The pathogenesis of rheumatoid arthritis (RA) is incompletely understood, but significant progress has been made in understanding the mechanisms which underlie the inflammation and joint destruction that characterize the disease. A better understanding of the contribution from T cells, B cells, cytokines and osteoclasts in the disease process has led to the development of therapeutics that have revolutionized the management of rheumatoid arthritis. Although cytokines are capable of inducing many of the *systemic* effects of arthritis such as weight loss, fever and fatigue, we will focus on the *local* effects of cytokines on synovial tissue. Table 2.1 lists the cells and mechanisms likely to be implicated in RA.

2.1 **T cells**

T cells become activated by antigen-presenting cells such as dendritic cells. These specialized cells process antigen (e.g. citrullinated self-peptides, see below) and present it to T cell receptors. Antigen

Table 2.1 Cells, cytokines and mechanisms implicated in the pathogenesis of rheumatoid arthritis

Cells	T cells	Enhancing disease through production of cytokines
Cells	B cells	Enhancing disease through production of immune complexes and cytokines
Cells	Macrophages	Enhancing disease through production of cytokines
Cells	Fibroblasts	Enhancing disease through production of cytokines and prolongation of T cell survival
Cells	Regulatory T cells	Resolution of inflammation by anti inflammatory cytokines to inhibit function of active immune cells
Cytokines	Pro-inflammatory mediators	Enhancing disease through local inflammatory cell proliferation, release of matrix metallaproteinases (MMPs) and angiogenesis
Cytokines	Anti-inflammatory mediators	Resolution of inflammation through inhibition of local inflammatory cell proliferation, release of MMPs and inhibiting cell signalling pathways
Mechanisms	Angiogenesis	Enhancing disease by supporting local inflammatory cell survival with oxygen and nutrients; local oedema
Mechanisms	Articular and bone destruction	Increased activity of MMPs in cartilage and osteoclasts on bone and cartilage

presentation occurs in association with cell surface glycoproteins known as major histocompatibility complexes, MHC (also known as human leucocyte antigens HLA). MHC proteins are coded on chromosome 6 in the loci HLA-DP, DQ and DR and are of two basic types: MHC class I is found on all nucleated cells and class II is restricted to B cells, activated T cells, macrophages and inflamed vascular endothelium.

T$_H$ cells recognize antigen in the presence of MHC class II, and a nearby accessory molecule CD4 (cluster differentiation 4) increases cell binding and signalling. T$_C$ cells, on the other hand, use MHC class I and CD8 to enhance cell binding and activation. These first T cell signals are *antigen-specific*. T cell activation is regulated through the requirement for a co-stimulatory signal (signal 2) resulting from binding of the CD28 protein on T cells with ligands (CD80/86) present on antigen-presenting cells. Activation occurs only in the presence of *both* signals. T cells may also express the protein CTLA4 that binds to CD80/86 without providing a co-stimulatory signal. The absence of dual signal leads to T cell anergy. The fusion protein abatacept acts by blocking co-stimulation (signal 2) by mimicking the action of CTLA4, thereby inhibiting T cell activation and expansion. (See Figure 2.1).

The possible importance of T cells in the pathogenesis of RA is suggested by the presence of activated CD4+ T cell infiltrates and T cell-derived cytokines in the synovial tissue of patients, and the

Figure 2.1 T cell signalling and activation

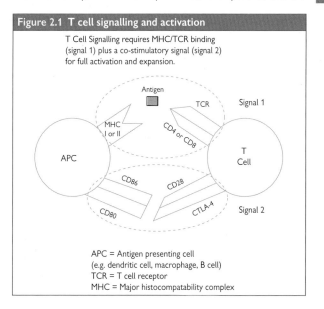

T Cell Signalling requires MHC/TCR binding (signal 1) plus a co-stimulatory signal (signal 2) for full activation and expansion.

APC = Antigen presenting cell
(e.g. dendritic cell, macrophage, B cell)
TCR = T cell receptor
MHC = Major histocompatability complex

association between RA and HLA-DR4 and -DR1 alleles that contain a shared amino acid motif in the antigen binding-site, commonly known as the shared epitope. Activated T cells persist in the rheumatoid joint as a result of local accumulation and local proliferation generated by cytokine and chemokine release. Interactions between adhesion molecules (including integrins, VCAM-1, ELAM-1 and LFA-1) expressed on venular endothelium in activated synovium causes non-specific trafficking of memory T cells into the synovial compartment. However, they are also likely to persist due to failure of the normal clearance such as cell migration and programmed cell death (apoptosis) which is inhibited by a number of mechanisms, including the effects of synovial fibroblasts. Treatments targeted at T cells, such as ciclosporin, abatacept, lymphoid irradiation and thoracic duct drainage, have all been shown to have beneficial effects in RA.

CD4+ T cells are known to be divided into at least three separate T-helper cell subsets, T_H1, T_H2 and T_H17. Each lineage displays a characteristic cytokine-producing profile and rheumatoid arthritis is characterized by an imbalance of these CD4+ T cell sub populations. T_H17 cells are the dominant cell population in RA, producing the cytokine interleukin -17 (IL-17). This potent pro-inflammatory cytokine is responsible for the induction of other major inflammatory cytokines such as IL-1, IL-6 and TNFα. In addition to its inflammatory role, IL-17 induces release of matrix metalloproteinases to degrade cartilage, and to osteoclast activation, leading to bone erosion. Animal models have shown that IL-17 deficiency protects against the development of collagen-induced arthritis (CIA). Table 2.2 lists the functions of activated T cells in RA.

Activated T cells are therefore involved in the development and persistence of joint inflammation (synovitis) and in bony and cartilage destruction. Regulatory T cells (CD4+CD25+), on the other hand, home to the site of inflammation and could act locally to resolve the inflammation. Their action is probably mediated through release of IL-10 and/or transforming growth factor beta (TGFβ). Their potential role in enhancing the resolution of inflammation in RA is the subject of considerable current research interest.

Table 2.2 Functions of activated T cells in RA
Induction of pro-inflammatory cytokines (e.g. IL-6, IL-7 and TNFα) to enlist and coordinate T cell, B cell and macrophage recruitment
Activation of synovial fibroblasts and osteoclasts to erode cartilage and bone
B cell proliferation and therefore antibody production
Release of metalloproteinases to degrade cartilage

2.2 B lymphocytes

The success of rituximab, a B cell-depleting agent, in RA has confirmed a likely role for the B cell in pathogenesis. The B cell is not only capable of autoantibody production, but also cytokine release, antigen presentation and modulation of T cells. The most crucial role is likely to be the development of autoantibodies such as directed to IgG molecules (rheumatoid factor, RF) and cyclic citrullinated peptides (ACPA). Serological testing for RF is complicated by its modest sensitivity and specificity and its prevalence in other inflammatory and infective conditions (see Chapter 3). ACPA promise earlier and more accurate diagnosis with, crucially, a greater specificity (up to 95%) than RF, although the sensitivity of 67% indicates that 1/3 of patients are negative as seen with RF. ACPA and RF correlate with greater disease activity/radiographic progression and appear before the onset of disease. They may therefore be of some use in early disease in targeting more aggressive therapy to those at particular risk of more severe disease. This suggests a role for screening those at risk of developing the disease (e.g. with a strong family history), and identifying patients at an early stage to offer aggressive intervention.

The citrullination of self-peptides occurs in other diseases (e.g. multiple sclerosis), but the subsequent development of antibodies appears to be specific to RA. It is not clear whether ACPA are directly involved in pathogenesis, contribute to ongoing inflammatory activity or are simply by-products of the inflammatory process. Several studies have reported an association between ACPA production and the genetic profile conferring risk of developing RA (known as the shared epitope in the MHC molecule -see above). In addition, cigarette smoking promotes the citrullination of self peptides and has been associated with the development of ACPA. It is possible that citrullinated peptides are processed by antigen-presenting cells with the high-risk HLA-DR shared epitope and are presented to T cells. The resultant T cell activation and expansion leads to cell-mediated immunity against citrullinated antigens, whilst reactive B cells secrete ACPA (see Figure 2.2). Indeed, recent evidence indicates that ectopic lymphoid structures within RA synovium are functional and able to generate such autoantibodies.

2.3 Macrophages

Tissue macrophages are derived from circulating monocytes. Both cell types are important in RA, with effects on initiating and perpetuating inflammation, promoting adhesion and migration of leukocytes,

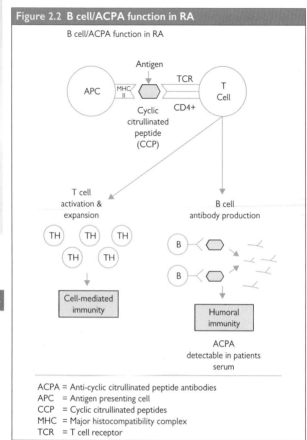

Figure 2.2 B cell/ACPA function in RA

B cell/ACPA function in RA

T cell
activation &
expansion

B cell
antibody production

Cell-mediated
immunity

Humoral
immunity

ACPA
detectable in patients
serum

ACPA = Anti-cyclic citrullinated peptide antibodies
APC = Antigen presenting cell
CCP = Cyclic citrullinated peptides
MHC = Major histocompatibility complex
TCR = T cell receptor

degradation of collagen matrix and angiogenesis. The macrophage is
the most important cell responsible for the production of TNFα in
the joint, but also produces a number of other cytokines including IL-1,
IL-6, IL-15, IL-18 and IL-23. Macrophages also present antigens to
T cells thereby driving the inflammatory process. They are activated
to produce pro-inflammatory cytokines by the presence of immune
complexes and T cells. In contrast to the adaptive immune response,
which targets specific antigens selectively, the innate immune response
regulates immune responsiveness in a more general fashion in
response to triggers that include lipopolysaccharides from bacterial
cell walls and naked DNA.

2.4 Fibroblasts

The most common cell found in normal synovial tissue of RA is the synovial fibroblast. These cells are morphologically distinct from healthy fibroblasts, as they express proto-oncogenes and anti-apoptotic molecules, and lack tumour suppressor genes. Synovial fibroblasts are effector cells, producing pro-inflammatory cytokines and chemo-ines and attracting activated inflammatory cells to the joint. In addition, they are directly responsible for cartilage erosion through the production of matrix-degrading enzymes.

2.5 Angiogenesis

Angiogenesis in synovial tissue is required to provide increased oxygen and nutrients for the local invasion of inflammatory cells, leading to further swelling and disease progression. Growth factors, cytokines, matrix metalloproteinases, matrix macromolecules, cell adhesion receptors, chemokines and chemokine receptors are all responsible for new capillary formation. Vascular endothelial growth factor (VEGF) also has a central role in angiogenesis and its action as a vascular permeability factor increases oedema in the joints. Targeting VEGF therefore offers a potential opportunity to modify the disease process. Other mediators which may also have an effect on angiogenesis include high mobility group box 1 (HMGB1). HMGB1 is a nuclear protein involved in chromatin architecture and regulation of transcription, but when it is released from macrophages in response to TNFα, it acts as a pro-inflammatory mediator. High levels have been found in synovial fluid from patients with RA, and RA in animal models can be significantly improved by neutralising the effects of this HMGB1.

2.6 Inflammatory mediators

Table 2.3 lists the key cytokines involved in RA. TNFα is of primary importance in the pathogenesis of RA, and for many patients, probably represents the dominant cytokine. It is present in high concentrations in both synovial fluid and rheumatoid synovium and through its widespread actions is responsible for key pathological processes. TNFα is also responsible for the systemic effects and weight loss seen in very active disease. Inhibition with anti-TNF biologic therapies (adalimumab, certolizumab, etanercept, infliximab) induces a rapid clinical response in up to 70% of patients with a sustained reduction in inflammatory cytokines and the acute phase response (see Chapter 6). IL-6 is also prominent in the inflammatory hierarchy, and blocking the

Table 2.3 Key cytokines in rheumatoid arthritis

Cytokine	Cellular source	Main function
IL-1	Macrophages, B cells, synovial fibroblasts	Release of other cytokines, matrix metalloproteinases (MMP) and prostaglandins
IL-6	Macrophages, synovial fibroblasts, T and B cells	B and T cell proliferation, induction of CRP, neuroendocrine effects
IL-12	Activated macrophages and dendritic cells	T-cell activation and T_H1 differentiation.
IL-15	Macrophages	T-cell activation
IL-17	T_H17 cells, synovial fibroblasts	Cytokine and MMP release, osteoclast activation
IL-18	Macrophages	Release of cytokines, chemokines and adhesion molecules, osteoclast activation
IL-23	Activated macrophages and dendritic	Activates T_H17 cells to produce IL-17
IL-32	Activated T cells and macrophages	Release of IL-1β, TNFα and IL-18
TNFα	Macrophages, T cells, B cells, synovial fibroblasts	Cellular activation, cytokine, MMP and prostaglandin release
IL-33	Synovial fibroblasts and macrophages	Stimulation of mast cells to generate IL-1, IL-6 and TNFα

soluble IL-6 receptor with a monoclonal antibody, tocilizumab, shows promise in recent studies. IL-1 is highly expressed in RA synovium, and therapeutic targeting with anakinra is also available. IL-1 blockade appears less effective than TNFα inhibition, although no direct head-to-head comparative study has yet been performed. IL-17 is responsible for many of the characteristic features of RA. Blockade of IL-17 via antibodies or soluble IL-17 receptors can reduce symptoms of even established CIA (an animal model of human RA); anti-IL-17 monoclonal antibodies for clinical trial in humans are in development. Recent evidence also demonstrates that IL-33, expressed by RA synovial fibroblasts, stimulates mast cells to generate a spectrum of inflammatory cytokines. Neutralising antibodies to IL-33 have been shown to reduce the severity of CIA and therefore may represent a therapeutic strategy for RA.

2.7 Anti-inflammatory cytokines

Anti-inflammatory T_H2 cells produce IL-4 and IL-10 which are generally more associated with humoral immunity and atopic responses.

However in RA, there is a dominance of T_H1 and T_H17 cells and it therefore consistent that the incidence of atopy is actually reduced in RA. Both IL-4 and IL-10 reduce the expression of T_H1 cytokines, HLA-DR and co-stimulatory molecules by macrophages. IL10 also has an effect on B cell survival, proliferation, and antibody production. It blocks NF-κB activity, and is involved in the regulation of other cell signaling pathways.

2.8 Articular cartilage and bone destruction

Inflammation, cartilage and bone loss are closely linked. The rapid degradation of cartilage seen in RA is driven by matrix metalloproteinases (MMPs) which are derived from synovial fibroblasts, neutrophil polymorphs, and from chondrocytes within the cartilage itself. The biologic activity of MMPs is modulated by their natural inhibitors-TIMPs (tissue inhibitors of MMP) so the balance between these is potentially critical in determining the degree of joint destruction and makes them valid targets for developing new treatments. In addition to the action of MMPs, the deeper mineralized layer of cartilage adjacent to bone is eroded by activated osteoclasts which burrow beneath the cartilage. The combined assault on cartilage from its surface, base and from within, leads to its rapid destruction.

In RA, the normal tight balance between bone formation and bone resorption is lost, leading to osteopaenia and joint erosion. Osteoclasts are specialized bone-resorbing cells, typically derived from circulating monocytes, which, on entry into inflamed synovial tissue, are exposed to activating signals, including TNFα. The essential signals for osteoclast development are macrophage colony-stimulating factor (MCSF) and receptor activator of nuclear factor-κB ligand (RANKL), expressed by synovial fibroblasts and activated T cells. IL-1, IL-6, IL-17 and TNFα are present in rheumatoid synovium, and augment osteoclastogenesis by inducing RANKL (see Figure 2.3). Denosumab, a monoclonal antibody directed against RANKL, has been shown to increase bone mineral density in patients with post-menopausal osteoporosis, and may also have the potential, in combination with methotrexate, to reduce bone erosions in RA.

Recent studies have also highlighted dickkopf-1 (DKK-1) as a critical regulator of joint remodeling. DKK-1 is expressed by RA synovium in response to TNFα and inhibits wingless (wnt)-signalling. Reduced wnt signaling has two effects on bone modeling: i) a direct inhibition of osteoblast activation and bone formation and ii) an indirect augmentation of osteoclastogenesis by decreasing expression of osteoprotegerin (OPG), the endogenous inhibitor of RANKL. Elevated levels of DKK-1 are found in patients with RA, correlate with disease activity and have been shown to return to normal on treatment with anti-TNF therapy.

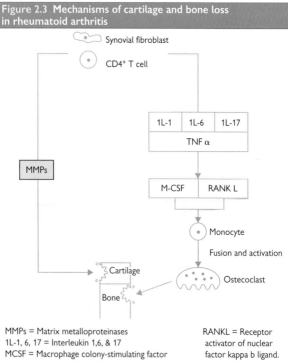

Figure 2.3 Mechanisms of cartilage and bone loss in rheumatoid arthritis

MMPs = Matrix metalloproteinases
1L-1, 6, 17 = Interleukin 1,6, & 17
MCSF = Macrophage colony-stimulating factor

RANKL = Receptor activator of nuclear factor kappa b ligand.

2.9 Summary

Rheumatoid arthritis results from immune system dysregulation at both cellular and humoral levels. Increasing understanding of the mechanisms underlying both the articular and systemic manifestations has led to the development of novel therapeutic strategies.

Further reading

McInnes IB, Schett G. Cytokines in the pathogenesis of rheumatoid arthritis. *Nat Rev Immunol.* 2007 Jun; **7**(6): 429–42.

Ospelt C, Gay S. The role of resident synovial cells in destructive arthritis. *Best Pract Res Clin Rheumatol.* 2008 Apr; **22**(2): 239–52.

Tarner IH, Müller-Ladner U, Gay S. Emerging targets of biologic therapies for rheumatoid arthritis. *Nat Clin Pract Rheumatol.* 2007 Jun; **3**(6): 336–45.

Toh ML, Miossec P. The role of T cells in rheumatoid arthritis: new subsets and new targets. *Curr Opin Rheumatol.* 2007 May; **19**(3): 284–8.

Chapter 3

Diagnosis and clinical features of rheumatoid arthritis

Raashid Luqmani, Maarten Boers and Theodore Pincus

Key points

- Patients with rheumatoid arthritis should be diagnosed as early as possible so that effective treatment can be initiated to prevent joint damage and comorbidities
- Any swelling or persistent (>3 weeks) pain and stiffness in multiple joint areas should prompt referral to a rheumatologist
- Typical joint patterns in RA include involvement of the metacarpophalangeal, metatarsophalangeal, wrist, and knee joints
- The more difficult differential diagnosis is fibromyalgia, which also can co-exist in 20% of cases
- Rheumatoid factor and ACPA testing are useful in making the diagnosis in patients with appropriate clinical features, and predicts poor radiological outcome, but >30% of patients are negative for these tests
- More than 40% of patients have normal ESR and CRP.

3.1 How do patients present?

Rheumatoid arthritis (RA) traditionally has been a simple diagnosis to make, based on a typical history and clinical findings. Until recent years, most patients were not seen until they had established disease, which had been regarded as relatively indolent in early years. However, it is now recognized that the natural history of rheumatoid arthritis is that of a potentially severe disease with functional declines and premature mortality. Therefore, currently, we aim to see patients as early as possible in their disease course, when classical findings may not be apparent.

Patients with early inflammatory arthritis, termed "early arthritis", present greater diagnostic complexity. 50–70% of individuals identified in population-based studies or early arthritis clinics appear to have a self-limited transient condition rather than a progressive disease. This matter complicates clinical decisions, and there is current disagreement over whether to offer empirical treatment with very low dose prednisolone to patients suspected of having a progressive inflammatory arthritis, analogous to empirical antibiotic treatment of patients with a suspected infection, although some authorities insist on a definitive diagnosis prior to any treatment.

The onset of RA may range from explosive to insidious. The most common presentation involves persistent discomfort over a period of several weeks affecting different joint areas, often in a migratory pattern. Patients usually experience pain in their small joints, often beginning in the feet, then spreading to involve wrists and metacarpophalangeal joints in a symmetrical distribution (Figure 3.1).

Patients generally complain of stiffness, or gelling, in the morning, so that it takes a little while to "loosen" their joints. However, morning stiffness also is reported by patients with fibromyalgia or osteoarthritis. Many patients try to deal with morning stiffness by measures such as taking a shower and slowing down their activities until their joints become more flexible. Swelling occurs in these joint areas, but patients may not be aware of this. General systemic features such as fatigue are common. In active disease, patients lose weight and may be feverish.

Examination of the joints can be difficult for a physician who is unfamiliar with looking after patients with arthritis. There are many joints to examine, and those who are not accustomed to assessing joints regularly may struggle with the findings. Patients with a suggestive history, with joint pain or stiffness persisting for more than 3 weeks, or with evidence of joint swelling should be referred to a rheumatologist. This allows the patient to be diagnosed more quickly and to start treatment when it has substantially greater potential to reduce the likelihood of long term damage.

In more advanced RA, it is easier to be confident in the joint examination, with tenderness, swelling, pain on motion, limited motion and/or deformity in affected joints. The physician should inspect and palpate the joints, and recognize limited motion, often using her/himself as a control subject. Swelling may be a subtle early feature characterized by loss of skin wrinkles around a joint, or the loss of dimples between joints, e.g., at the MCP joints (Figure 3.2). In more severe involvement, there may be a pronounced swelling that distorts the normal contours (Figure 3.3). A flexion deformity may be seen, because joint capsular tension is relieved by slight flexion, reducing the amount of pain felt by the patient (see Figure 3.4). Flexion contractures in the PIP joints or knees can be a useful feature to help establish a diagnosis.

Figure 3.1 Typical pattern of joint disease in RA

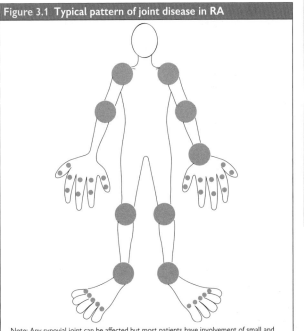

Note: Any synovial joint can be affected but most patients have involvement of small and medium sized joints as shown above.

Figure 3.2 Early RA in hands

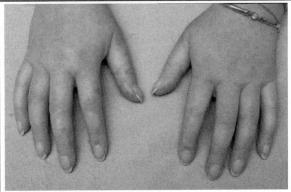

Note: Swelling may be a subtle early feature characterized by loss of skin wrinkles around a joint, or the loss of dimples between joints, e.g., at the MCP joints.

Figure 3.3 Moderate RA in hands

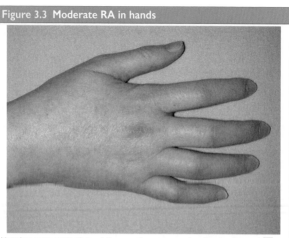

Note: In more severe involvement, there may be a pronounced swelling that distorts the normal contours – joints.

Figure 3.4 More advanced RA in hands

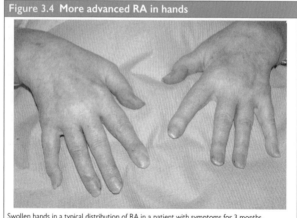

Swollen hands in a typical distribution of RA in a patient with symptoms for 3 months.

In older patients, the picture may be confused by the presence of osteoarthritic changes, particularly when there is bony swelling of the proximal interphalangeal joints (Figure 3.5). Joint enlargement may be seen in both inflammatory arthritis and OA, but careful palpation of these joints is helpful: in OA the joint line is hard and the swelling is an extension of the underlying joint margins; in RA, by contrast, the

Figure 3.5 OA in the hands

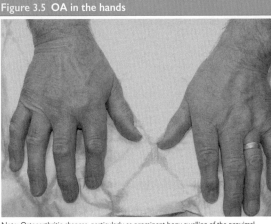

Note: Osteoarthritic changes, particularly as prominent bony swelling of the proximal interphalangeal joints.

swelling is soft, representing soft tissue or fluid in the joint. Palpation of the joint is also performed to determine whether or not the patient reports that the joint is tender. Tenderness is difficult to assess in the shoulder and hip, and sometimes other joints; pain on movement is an alternative assessment.

Less common forms of presentation may be seen, such as single large joint disease, e.g. shoulder or knee, or asymmetrical oligoarticular presentation. Older patients may have features of polymyalgia rheumatica – typically morning stiffness with shoulder and hip girdle discomfort, associated with weight loss, fatigue and lymphadenopathy. Often it is impossible to distinguish polymyalgia rheumatica from polymyalgic onset RA – some authors have suggested that PMR is a form of rheumatoid factor-negative RA. In practice, it is usual to institute treatment for PMR (typically 10–15 mg per day prednisolone.) If, despite improvement in their systemic symptoms, the patients develop small joint pain and swelling, this suggests that the diagnosis was actually "polymyalgic–onset" RA. A diagnosis of RA is reinforced by finding that the patient has a positive rheumatoid factor test, or ACPA, if available.

The American College of Rheumatology has published classification criteria for use in clinical studies (Table 3.1). These criteria serve as a useful checklist, but classification criteria are not the same as diagnostic criteria, and cannot be used to make a definitive diagnosis. For example, rheumatoid factor is present in low titre in some normal individuals, most of whom do not develop RA, and is not present at all in 30–40% of patients with definite RA.

Table 3.1 American College of Rheumatology classification of RA
• Morning stiffness for >1 hour
• Arthritis involving at least 3 joint areas
• Arthritis affecting hand joints
• Symmetrical distribution of arthritis
• Presence of rheumatoid nodules
• Presence of rheumatoid factor in blood tests
• Presence of bony erosions on X-rays
Data from the American College of Rheumatology http://www.rheumatology.org/publications/classification/ra/1987_revised_criteria_classification_ra.asp?aud=mem

3.2 What is the differential diagnosis?

The differential diagnosis with most common presentations of RA is limited, but can be very wide for unusual forms of presentation. Table 3.2 lists conditions which should be considered in patients with new arthritis. If one is unfamiliar with assessing joint disease, it is possible to mistake RA for OA; however, involvement of MCPs and PIPs, wrists, often also the MTPs, makes an inflammatory arthritis most likely. By contrast, patients with OA may complain of pain swelling and stiffness, but the pattern of joint involvement in generalised nodal OA is typically of the DIP and PIP joints; the base of the thumb is often affected (1st CMC joint) but not MCP joints and wrists.

3.3 What clues are there in the history and examination?

The most useful clue to the diagnosis of RA is detectable soft tissue joint swelling, with tenderness. Patients may have nodules, especially at sites of bony prominence such as the elbow. Patients often experience fatigue, and describe it as being like having "flu" all the time.

RA is characterized by persistence, and progression, though the rate of progression varies widely in different individual patients. The pain and stiffness are present every day. Diurnal variation is typically seen in morning stiffness, or "gelling". This may persist for hours, but is defined as lasting more than 30 minutes, before the patient feels that the joints are starting to become limber. This may involve a few or all of the affected joints, but not just one or two. In OA for example, patients often feel stiff on wakening, but this often resolves within 30 minutes.

Table 3.2 Common differential diagnosis of RA	
OA	Different pattern of distribution – involving PIPs/DIPs but sparing wrists. Beware some patients can have both conditions.
Polymyalgia rheumatica	Polymyalgia onset RA can appear to be identical to PMR – the appearance of pain and swelling in small and medium sized joints may distinguish it from true PMR.
Psoriatic arthritis	Look for evidence of skin, scalp, and buttock or nail psoriasis; asymmetric pattern, oligoarthritis, DIP joint involment, inflammation of whole finger and toe ('sausage toe').
Polyarticular gout	Tophi, not nodules are present; they are often very superficial and look pale, sometimes white, and may exude uric acid if the skin breaks over them. Chronic tophaceous gout in an elderly female on long term diuretics may be a presentation of gout.
Systemic lupus erythematosus	Younger women with SLE may present with polyarthritis, but have other disease features such as hair loss, mouth ulcers and rashes.
Reactive arthritis	Usually history suggests a recent infection, and the joint disease is asymmetrical often predominantly lower limb.
Post infectious arthritis	Most viral and bacterial infections can produce a polyarthritis in a pattern that appears to be RA and may meet classification criteria, including the presence of rheumatoid factor. Most will resolve in a matter of weeks. Parvovirus B19 is the most common cause.
Chronic Pain/ Fibromyalgia	Many people (women more than men) have chronic widespread pain or fibromyalgia. Thay may be referred to the rheumatologist for evaluation, particularly those 10–15% who have a weakly positive RF. Clinical examination does not reveal evidence of swelling or limited motion. It is important to remember that 20% of patients with RA will also have concominant fibromyalgia
Pyrophosphate arthropathy	In elderly patients with longstanding chondro-calcinosis involvement of the 2nd and 3rd MCP and wrists may cause confusion; the history is often helpful, describing episodic swelling of joints; clinical findings are more suggestive of degenerative joint disease.
Malignancy	If patients have a systemic presentation of disease, the excess weight loss, fever and fatigue may suggest an underlying cancer, although weight loss and fatigue may be severe in RA.

3.4 What investigations are helpful?

In typical cases, particularly those with established RA, further investigations are not required to make the diagnosis, which is usually obvious from the history and examination. Tests may be done to confirm the clinical suspicion of the diagnosis of RA, and as a way of supporting the clinical decision to treat patients. However, in early disease, the diagnosis may be quite difficult. Laboratory tests may be more helpful then, when patients themselves may express doubt about a clinical diagnosis and be reluctant to embark on what they might perceive as toxic therapy.

There are no laboratory tests that give absolute certainty of the diagnosis, and laboratory tests should not be used in isolation to make a diagnosis in patients who do not have any suggestive clinical features.

Testing for rheumatoid factor (RF) and/or ACPA is helpful. RF is more sensitive, i.e. present in 69% of patients, but found in 10–15% of the general population, whereas ACPA is more specific for RA, i.e., present in 67% of patients and in 3–4% of the general population. It is likely that ACPA may be involved in the pathogenesis of RA (see Chapter 2). However, it is important to emphasize that 1 in 3 patients with RA do not have positive test for RF. Severity of disease, in terms of radiographic progression, is worse for patients with RF, or ACPA or both. By contrast, there are only weak associations between RF or ACPA and functional disability, pain, or work disability.

A blood count typically shows anaemia of chronic disease; an elevated ESR or CRP indicates the presence of systemic inflammation. Routine biochemistry testing may show mildly abnormal liver function, due to the systemic inflammation of RA, but more commonly due to toxicity from non steroidal anti-inflammatory drugs (diclofenac is particularly likely to be responsible).

A chest X-ray is important to rule out other conditions (for example a malignancy) which might mimic RA; in some centres it is routine practice to perform a chest X-ray prior to starting methotrexate (the usual first-choice DMARD).

3.5 Imaging of joints: X-ray, Ultrasound and MRI

Early in the course of the disease, plain X-rays of the hands and feet are often normal. However, many patients with RF or ACPA-positive disease may have subtle abnormalities on presentation and this indicates a poor prognosis if these patients are not promptly treated. Over time, radiographic features of arthritis will develop in untreated patients and even in treated patients if control of inflammation is incomplete. Radiographic progression is the basis of so-called "disease-modifying anti-rheumatic drugs" (DMARDs), since their use has been documented to slow (retard) development of radiographic damage.

The earliest finding is soft tissue swelling and loss of bone density around the joints due to increased vascular supply to the inflamed area (periarticular osteoporosis) (see Figure 3.6). These changes may develop within a few weeks. Within months the bone around joints especially in the hands and forefeet, will erode because of the invasive destructive nature of the synovial pannus (erosions). Abnormalities are often first seen in the MTP joints of the feet. (see Figure 3.7) In addition, cartilage is lost resulting in narrowing, and eventual disappearance of joint space. Over several years, a joint may become so damaged that it is completely destroyed, and the two ends of bone may fuse together in very advanced cases (ankylosis). Figure 3.8 shows a patient with very advanced destructive disease affecting the shoulders.

The availability of musculoskeletal ultrasound means that joints can be imaged in greater detail, revealing the presence of soft tissue swelling, increased vascular supply to the joints (on colour Doppler) and also shows the presence of erosions more commonly than can be seen on X-ray (Figure 3.9). However, it is not entirely

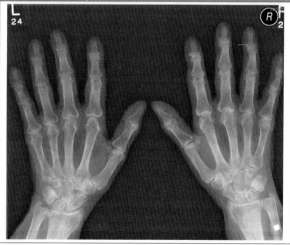

Figure 3.6 X-ray of a patient with early RA who has marked periarticular osteoporosis and soft tissue swelling around the MCP and PIP joints

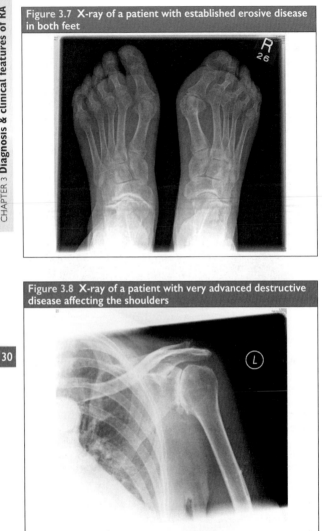

Figure 3.7 **X-ray of a patient with established erosive disease in both feet**

Figure 3.8 **X-ray of a patient with very advanced destructive disease affecting the shoulders**

Figure 3.9 Doppler ultrasound to show synovitis in RA

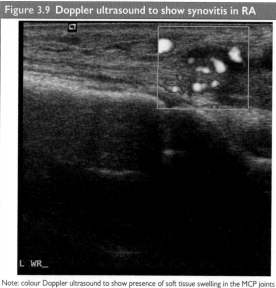

L WR_

Note: colour Doppler ultrasound to show presence of soft tissue swelling in the MCP joints increased vascular supply to the joints (on) and also shows the presence of erosions 6 times more commonly than can be seen on X-ray.

clear that 'erosions' seen on ultrasound scans long before they are apparent on X-ray indicate the same phenomena. It is possible that ultrasound is showing what may be potentially reversible bony changes, whilst X-ray erosions suggest well-established, irreversible damage.

Magnetic resonance imaging (MRI) of joints yields impressive, high-quality images (Figure 3.10). However, the prognostic significance of MRI findings or how well abnormalities seen on MRI are correlated with clinical findings and with X-ray progression of disease remain uncertain.

Ultrasound and MRI examinations of joints are not routinely available and should continue to be regarded as research tools. Emerging findings from specialized research settings will provide further information concerning their possible clinical usefulness.

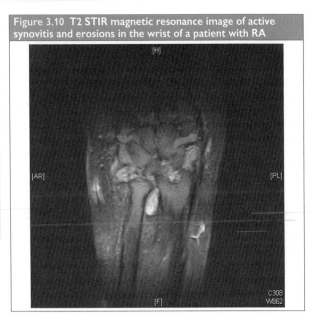

Figure 3.10 T2 STIR magnetic resonance image of active synovitis and erosions in the wrist of a patient with RA

3.6 Can we offer prognostic information?

For best management of RA, it would be very valuable to know which patients were likely to do worse, and which were likely to have a milder course of disease, so that perhaps, in future with more effective drugs, we could target patients according to need, rather than giving them all the same regimen as happens at present. Factors associated with poor outcome in terms of radiographic progression include: the presence of rheumatoid factor and or ACPA, cigarette smoking and the presence of the shared epitope of HLA class II (see Chapter 1). However, these epidemiologic data refer to groups of patients, and decisions concerning the level of intensity of therapies are generally based on the clinical findings and course in individual patients.

Most patients with RA have a natural history of progressive disease. Poor function, and the presence of co-morbidity and joint damage at presentation are significant markers of poor prognosis,. Therefore, it is desirable to minimize disease activity using single or combination DMARD therapy early to control inflammation as well as possible.

3.7 Extra-articular disease in RA

This is discussed in Chapter 8.

Further reading

Aletaha D, Landewe R, Karonitsch T, Bathon J, Boers M, Bombardier C, et al; EULAR; ACR. Reporting disease activity in clinical trials of patients with rheumatoid arthritis: EULAR/ACR collaborative recommendations. *Arthritis Rheum*. 2008 Oct 15;**59**(10):1371–7.

Deighton C, O'Mahony R, Tosh J, Turner C, Rudolf M; Guideline Development Group. Management of rheumatoid arthritis: summary of NICE guidance. *BMJ*. 2009 Mar 16;338:b702. doi: 10.1136/bmj.b702.

Luqmani R, Hennell S, Estrach C, Basher D, Birrell F, Bosworth A, et al; British Society for Rheumatology; British Health Professionals in Rheumatology Standards, Guidelines and Audit Working Group. British Society for Rheumatology and British Health Professionals in Rheumatology guideline for the management of rheumatoid arthritis (after the first 2 years). *Rheumatology* (Oxford). 2009 Apr;**48**(4):436–9.

Chapter 4

Disease assessment and monitoring patients for follow up

Theodore Pincus and Raashid Luqmani

Key points

- It is important to use a quantitative clinical measure, not just a laboratory test at each patient visit in order to evaluate disease status
- The aim of treatment is to achieve remission, ideally guided by a quantitative index
- Be aware of comorbidities, which are common in patients with RA
- Record information in a structured format and include a flowsheet so that the change in disease status can readily be recognized.

Assessment of patients with rheumatoid arthritis (RA) is complex. No single "gold standard" measure, such as blood pressure in the case of hypertension or haemoglobin A1c in diabetes mellitus, is available for diagnosis, prognosis, monitoring and documenting change in status in all patients with RA. The 2 major serologic tests for RA, rheumatoid factor and anti-cyclic citrullinated peptide (ACPA) antibodies, and the 2 major acute phase reactants for inflammatory activity, erythrocyte sedimentation rate (ESR) and C-reactive protein (CRP), are abnormal in 60%–70% of patients with RA. Therefore, more than one-third of individual patients with progressive RA have normal values for each test, and more than one-sixth have normal values for all these laboratory tests.

Assessment which includes quantitative information can be applied to provide "tight" control of RA, with better outcomes. Patients should undergo regular quantitative assessment of disease status, beyond laboratory tests. A core data set of 7 measures has been developed for use in clinical trials and in clinical practice (Table 4.1).

	ACR	DAS28	CDAI	RAPID3
		Table 4.1 Indices Based on Core Data Set for RA		
Number of tender joints	✓	$0.56 \times$ sq rt (TJC28)	0–28	–
Number of swollen joints	✓	$0.28 \times$ sq rt (SJC28)	0–28	–
MD global	✓	–	0–10	–
ESR or CRP	✓	$0.70 \times \ln$ (ESR)	–	–
Patient function	✓	–	–	0–10
Patient pain	✓	–	–	0–10
Patient global	✓	$0.014 \times$ PTGL	0–10	0–10
TOTAL	✓	0–10	0–76	0–30

From these 7 measures, it is possible to derive indices consisting of a smaller number of measures, which are used in clinical trials and standard clinical care. Available indices include the disease activity score (DAS28), clinical disease activity index (CDAI), and the routine assessment of patient index data (RAPID3), which consists of only patient self-report measures. The measures and indices are discussed briefly below:

Joint count. The classical joint count scores 66–68 joints for swelling, tenderness, limited motion, pain on motion, and deformity (Table 4.2). The Ritchie index assesses 52 joints for joint tenderness, grouping proximal interphalangeal (PIP) and metacarpophalangeal (MCP) joints. A 28 joint count includes 10 PIP, 10 MCP, 2 wrist, 2 elbow, 2 shoulder, and 2 knee joints. A 28 joint count does not require undressing the patient, is widely used in clinical trials, and is the basis of a DAS28.

Joint examination is the most specific measure for diagnosis and monitoring of patients with rheumatoid arthritis (RA). However, a formal joint count is relatively poorly reproducible, and no more (generally less) efficient than other core data set measures to recognize differences between active and control treatments in clinical trials. Most rheumatologists do not perform formal joint counts at most visits, except in clinical research or if required for therapies, such as biological therapies, despite directives over a half-century. A careful joint examination without an exact count may be sufficient to guide clinical decisions, particularly if patient questionnaire data are available for quantitative monitoring of patient status.

Laboratory tests. Traditional emphasis in medical practice has been focused on laboratory tests, which are essential in the management of acute diseases, and can be useful in the management of chronic diseases.

As noted, tests for rheumatoid factor, ACPA, ESR and CRP are abnormal in 60%–70% of patients with RA, and therefore normal in at least 30% of patients with progressive disease. Laboratory tests can be helpful in many patients, but if used in isolation, will miss a substantial number of patients who appear to need more aggressive treatment. Furthermore, laboratory tests may not change despite substantial changes in patient status, and are of limited value in patient assessment and monitoring. Laboratory testing of cell counts and biochemistry, however, is an essential component of monitoring for potential toxicities of DMARD therapy (see Chapter 5).

Patient questionnaire measures. Patient questionnaires have become increasingly prominent in the management of RA since their introduction 30 years ago. Physical function assessed on a patient questionnaire, rather than a laboratory test or radiograph, is usually the most significant predictor of outcomes in RA, including work disability, cost, and premature mortality. The classical patient questionnaire in RA is the health assessment questionnaire (HAQ), which addresses 20 activities of daily living (ADL), as well as queries about aids and devices, and help from another person. Performance of the 20 ADL is rated by the patient on a 0-3 scale: "without any difficulty (=0)," "with some difficulty (=1)," "with much difficulty (=2)," or "unable to do (=3)," and classified into 8 categories. The HAQ disability index (HAQ-DI) is the mean of the 8 highest scores among 2 or 3 ADL in each category, with scores for the category raised by one unit if aids, devices or help are needed.

The complexities of scoring the HAQ in usual care have led to abbreviated versions with 10 activities, which are easily scored as the simple mean of 10, including the HAQ-II and multidimensional HAQ (MDHAQ). The HAQ-II has superior measurement properties, while the MDHAQ includes an item from each of 8 categories of the HAQ, as well as 2 more advanced activities – walk 2 miles or 3 kilometers, and participate in sports or recreation as you would like. It is more accurate for the patient to complete a questionnaire by self-report than for a health professional to participate in completion of the questionnaire.

Global measures. Physician and patient estimates of global status usually are highly correlated, because physicians gain most of their estimates from patients, although the scores are occasionally disparate. The traditional 1–4 scale, known as American Rheumatism Association (ARA) functional class, is an excellent descriptor of physician estimate of clinical status, but insensitive to change, because patients may remain in class 2 or 3 despite extensive change in status. A 0–10 global estimate can be scored as quickly as a 1–4 estimate, but is more sensitive

Table 4.2 Comparison of joints included in various standard joint counts			
Joint	66/68 joints	Ritchie Index	28 joints
Temporomandibular	+	+*	
Sternoclavicular	+	+*	
Acromioclavicular	+	+*	
Shoulder	+	+	+
Elbow	+	+	+
Wrist	+	+	+
Metacarpophalangeal		+	
First	+		+
Second	+		+
Third	+		+
Fourth	+		+
Fifth	+		+
Proximal interphalangeal		+	
First	+		+
Second	+		+
Third	+		+
Fourth	+		+
Fifth	+		+
Distal interphalangeal			
Second	+		
Third	+		
Fourth	+		
Fifth	+		
Hip	+#	+	
Knee	+	+	+
Ankle	+	+	
Talocalcaneal		+	
Tarsus	+	+	
Metatarsophalangeal		+	
First	+		
Second	+		
Third	+		
Fourth	+		
Fifth	+		

Table 4.2 *(Contd.)*			
Joint	66/68 joints	Ritchie Index	28 joints
Proximal interphalangeal (toe)			
First	+		
Second	+		
Third	+		
Fourth	+		
Fifth	+		
# Assessed for tenderness only; * Right and left joint assessed together			

to detect a change in status. Indeed, global scales appear to be as effective in distinguishing active from control treatments in clinical trials as any core data set measure.

Patient global estimate, completed on self-report as a 0–10 scale, is a similarly useful measure. A written or computer-scored patient self-report of global status is a considerably more useful measure than a patient response to a query by a health professional of "how are you doing?" A 0–10 scale (with 0.5 increments) in 21 numbered circles appears to provide similar results to the traditional 10-cm line, rendering it possible to score without a ruler.

Indices to measure RA. The American College of Rheumatology (ACR) core data set measures have been used to describe response criteria based on % improvement from baseline at 20%, 50%, and 70% levels for tender and swollen joint counts plus 3 of the other 5 measures, as "ACR20," "ACR50," or "ACR70" responses. These response criteria have been useful in clinical trials but do not provide an absolute score to assess status and change in clinical practice.

The most extensively used index in clinical practice has been the DAS28, which was developed through discriminant analysis of values of measures at visits at which clinicians changed disease-modifying anti-rheumatic drugs (DMARDs). The DAS28 consists of 4 measures (28 swollen joint count, 28 tender joint count, ESR or CRP, and patient estimate of global status – scored 0–10). Levels of activity include high (>5.1), moderate (3.2–5.1), low (2.6–3.19) and remission (<2.6), and improvement criteria based on these levels have been described (Table 4.3). Some reports have suggested that more stringent criteria for remission may be needed. A calculator or a computer is required for a DAS; on-line calculators and software programs which include DAS calculators are available.

The clinical disease activity index (CDAI), was developed to overcome complexities of the DAS28, in not requiring a calculator or computer, or a laboratory test, which often is not available at the time of a patient visit. The CDAI includes a swollen joint count, tender

Table 4.3 EULAR improvement criteria based on DAS levels

EULAR improvement criteria for DAS28

Disease activity level	DAS28 at endpoint	Improvement in DAS28 from baseline		
		>1.2	>0.6 and ≤1.2	≤0.6
"low"	≤3.2	good	moderate	none
"moderate"	>3.2 and ≤5.1	moderate	moderate	none
"high"	>5.1	moderate	none	none

Fransen and van Riel, *Clin Exp Rheumatol* 23:S-93-S99, 2005

joint count, patient estimate of global status, and physician estimate of global status, scored 0–76: 0–28 for each of two joint counts and 0–10 for each of two global estimates. The CDAI has been found to be as informative as DAS28 in clinical trials and clinical care.

An index composed of only the 3 patient-reported Core Data Set measures for physical function, pain and global status – routine assessment of patient index data 3 (RAPID3) distinguishes active from control treatments as effectively as DAS28 or CDAI in clinical trials and is correlated significantly with these indices. RAPID3 is scored 0-30, 0-10 for each of the 3 questionnaire responses; the 0-30 scale may be divided by 3 for a 0-10 total score, but 0-30 is simpler. Levels of severity include high (>12 on a 0-30 scale), moderate (6.01-12 on a 0-30 scale, low (3.01-6 on a 0-30 scale, and remission (≤3 on a 0-30 scale).

4.1 Imaging studies

Radiographs are important to document joint damage. Current practice is directed to prevent radiographic abnormalities, in contrast to traditional teaching 20 years ago to treat with DMARD's only after there was evidence of radiographic damage. A classical 1–4 radiographic scale was described in 1949 by Steinbrocker, which is correlated significantly with other measures, but not sensitive to detect changes over time. Excellent detailed quantitative scoring systems have been developed by Larsen and Sharp, with modifications by van der Heijde, Rau, and others. However, these quantitative scales are complex to score and are rarely used except in clinical trials and studies.

Radiographs provide optimal documentation of joint destruction, but are far weaker predictors of work disability and premature mortality than functional status. Radiographs are less sensitive to identify abnormalities than magnetic resonance imaging (MRI) and ultrasound, which, however, are still regarded primarily as research tools to describe the "natural history" of RA. One explanation for the poor prognostic capacity of radiographs in RA clinical research may be that most research studies of radiographs involve the hands and feet, which appear less important in the prognosis of work disability or survival than large joints such as knees, hips, and shoulders.

4.2 **Approach to patient monitoring**

A traditional approach that patients should achieve moderate improvement has been replaced by a goal of as near to remission as possible for all patients. Nonetheless, some patients have substantial joint damage and/or have somatization or fibromyalgia, which may limit therapeutic responses. As noted, a quantitative index can be used to guide therapy. Some patients are happy to maintain status and not have worsening. The clinician and patient must agree on common treatment goals, which may vary considerably among different individual patients.

Patients should be seen as often as appears necessary, with frequent visits in the initial phase until patients achieve stability, then less often, such as semi-annual or annual review, but with additional visits if there is deterioration. Quantitative data should be collected at each visit, including regular laboratory tests for liver and renal function, complete blood counts, and ESR or CRP. Monitoring using a HAQ by mail has been successfully implemented, and may be an increasingly used future strategy, particularly where there is a shortage of rheumatologists.

If patients have active disease, it is important to try to understand why. Have there been any changes in their normal routine or new physical, emotional or medical stress? For example, if they had recently started to do more gardening as a result of improvement in their disease, this could have worsened the hand arthritis; bereavement, divorce and other emotional events can trigger episodes of active arthritis; infection, surgery or other medical conditions such as myocardial infarction or other active acute co-morbidity could exacerbate the disease. If these factors were not present or cannot be changed, the underlying therapy may require escalation to regain control of disease; this may require higher doses of the same therapy, additional DMARD therapy or a change of therapy, depending on how they have previously responded.

4.3 **Other health professionals**

Although pharmacologic therapy is the mainstay of care for patients with RA, attention to many other matters is important to achieve good outcomes. Other health professionals, including other physicians and surgeons can be extremely important (see Chapter 7). A physical therapist can guide an exercise program, particularly with evidence that exercise has positive effects not only on general fitness, but also improves musculoskeletal function in patients with arthritis.

An occupational therapist can assist patients with functional status in activities of daily living. Social workers can be helpful with family and interpersonal matters. Rehabilitation counselors can be effective in the preservation of work status.

The rheumatologist must also be mindful of complications of RA and drug toxicities in monitoring patients with RA (Table 4.4). Comorbidities which may be associated with disease pathophysiology and (less often) with therapies. These are discussed more extensively in Chapter 8.

Table 4.4 Complications of RA and drug toxicity to be reviewed in routine monitoring

Complication	Clues
Cervical cord compression	Patients may have new or worsening neck pain, with long tract signs in the legs, or just have stiff legs without evidence of active arthritis
Ischaemic heart disease	NSAIDs are implicated as a risk factor, but RA itself increases the likelihood of myocardial infarction. As a routine, patients should have other traditional risk factors for IHD assessed and minimised e.g. encourage them to stop smoking, check and treat high blood pressure, check blood glucose at least e.g. annually, measure cholesterol annually
Anaemia	Most patients with RA become anaemic during the course of their disease; it may be due to uncontrolled disease activity (anaemia of chronic disease, which is normochromic and normocytic and does not respond to oral iron); drugs such as NSAIDs commonly cause GI blood loss, unless co-prescribed with a proton pump inhibitor or H2 antagonist
Abnormal liver function tests	Patients receiving NSAIDs and DMARD therapy (usually methotrexate and or leflunomide) may develop abnormal LFTs- for NSAIDs, the drug should be stopped; for MTX and LFN, LFTs are commonly abnormal and within twice the upper limit of normal it is common and safe practice to continue treatment
Thrombocytopenia	Usually secondary to DMARDs; may require temporary or permanent change in therapy; thrombocytopenia in long standing RA may be a feature of Felty's syndrome- such patients will have neutropenia and splenomegaly

Table 4.4 (Contd.)	
Complication	Clues
Neutropenia	Usually secondary to DMARDs; may require temporary or permanent change in therapy; neutropenia in long standing RA may be a feature of Felty's syndrome- such patients will have thrombocytopenia and splenomegaly
Joint failure	With long standing disease or very aggressive destructive disease, joints may start to fail; early review by an orthopaedic surgeon specialized in managing RA is recommended

Further reading

Aletaha D, Smolen J: The simplified disease activity index (SDAI) and the clinical disease activity index (CDAI): a review of their usefulness and validity in rheumatoid arthritis. Clin Exp Rheumatol 2005; **23**: S100–S108.

Fuchs HA, Brooks RH, Callahan LF, Pincus T: A simplified twenty-eight joint quantitative articular index in rheumatoid arthritis. Arthritis Rheum 1989; **32**: 531–7.

Hewlett S, Kirwan J, Pollock J, et al.: Patient initiated outpatient follow up in rheumatoid arthritis: six year randomised controlled trial. Br J Med J 2005; **330**: 171–4.

Pincus T, Yazici Y, Sokka T: Quantitative measures of rheumatic diseases for clinical research versus standard clinical care: differences, advantages and limitations. Best Pract Res Clin Rheumatol 2007; **21**(4): 601–28.

Pincus T, Yazici Y, Bergman M: A practical guide to scoring a Multi-Dimensional Health Assessment Questionnaire (MDHAQ) and Routine Assessment of Patient Index Data (RAPID) scores in 10–20 seconds for use in standard clinical care, without rulers, calculators, websites or computers. Best Pract Res Clin Rheumatol 2007; **21**(4): 755–87.

Prevoo MLL, van't Hof MA, Kuper HH, van Leeuwen MA, van de Putte LBA, van Riel PLCM: Modified disease activity scores that include twenty-eight-joint counts: Development and validation in a prospective longitudinal study of patients with rheumatoid arthritis. Arthritis Rheum 1995; **38**: 44–8.

Chapter 5

Drug therapy - small molecules

David L Scott and Gabrielle Kingsley

> **Key points**
>
> - Analgesics and NSAIDs reduce pain in RA and decrease joint tenderness and stiffness; neither type of drug modifies the course of RA
> - DMARDs reduce joint inflammation, improve function and reduce the progression of joint damage
> - Glucocorticoids help to control active RA and reduce the progression of joint damage but long-term toxicity substantially limits their value
> - Conventional treatments suppress but do not cure RA

5.1 Managing rheumatoid arthritis

Drugs used to treat rheumatoid arthritis are categorized traditionally into four main groups. The first group comprises drugs which primarily relieve symptoms such as analgesics and non-steroidal anti-inflammatory drugs. The second group consists of the disease modifying anti-rheumatic drugs which, in addition to relieving symptoms, aim to alter the outcome of the disease. The third group is glucocorticoids now also considered disease-modifying drugs. A fourth group is that of the biologic agents. The first three groups, which may be termed collectively 'small molecules' are considered sequentially in this chapter, the fourth in the next chapter.

Drugs are also used in rheumatoid arthritis to treat complications and co-morbidities, for example cardiovascular risk and osteoporosis; these drugs are also discussed in Chapter 8.

5.2 Symptom management

5.2.1 Available drugs and indications

Pain and the symptoms of joint inflammation such as joint tenderness and morning stiffness require symptomatic treatment. Both simple analgesics and non-steroidal anti-inflammatory drugs (NSAIDs) can be used to reduce some or all of these symptoms (Table 5.1). NSAIDs have the advantage of reducing both pain and symptoms of joint inflammation. However they are also more likely to result in adverse events.

5.2.2 Analgesics

Simple analgesics are useful for controlling pain in all patients with inflammatory arthritis. They span paracetamol (also termed acetaminophen), weak opioids, tramadol and combinations of paracetamol and weak opioids. The evidence base supporting their use is weak because treatment effects are small. This limitation is counterbalanced by extensive experience of using them in clinical practice. As a consequence they are widely recommended. However, few patients' symptoms are relieved by analgesics alone.

Paracetamol (acetaminophen) is widely used. At the recommended dosage (up to 1 g qds) there are few side effects, although high doses have been reported to cause dyspepsia and there is evidence of increased risk of upper gastrointestinal tract ulceration compared to placebo. However, it is usually well tolerated by patients with peptic ulcers, although higher doses (4g per day) may be as toxic as NSAIDs. Its interactions with other treatments are not a problem. Large overdoses result in liver damage. However, its efficacy is limited and it has a short half-life; consequently patients generally must take 6 to 8 tablets daily to achieve analgesic benefits.

Weak opioids such as codeine and dihydrocodeine are widely used. Dihydrocodeine has about twice the potency of codeine. Opioids show a ceiling effect for analgesia with higher doses resulting in progressively more adverse effects, particularly nausea, vomiting and constipation.

Tramadol is a synthetic, centrally acting analgesic, with some opioid properties. It causes less constipation than opiates. Dependence is not a clinically relevant problem. To be fully effective, tramadol must be given at a dose of 50–100 mg every 4–6 hours. A slow release formulation can be useful if night pain is a particular problem. Adverse effects include headache, dizziness and somnolence; these may preclude its use when patients must be mentally alert in the day.

Table 5.1 Main analgesics and non-steroidal anti-inflammatory drugs (NSAIDs)	
Analgesics	NSAIDs
Paracetamol (acetaminophen)	Ibuprofen
Codeine and Dihydrocodeine	Diclofenac
Tramadol	Naproxen
Paracetamol/Codeine (Co-codamol)	Celecoxib (COX-II Specific)
Paracetamol/Dihydrocodeine(Co-dydramol)	Etoricoxib (COX-II Specific)

Paracetamol (acetaminophen) is often combined with a weak opiate in a single tablet. Examples include combinations with codeine (co-codamol, vicodin) and dihydrocodeine (co-dydramol, hydrocodon). These compound drugs have the same effects and adverse reactions as individual drugs.

A novel approach to managing chronic pain is the use of transdermal opiate patches containing buprenorphine or fentanyl. Transdermal fentanyl has been tested in rheumatoid arthritis and large joint osteoarthritis and shown to improve pain control and quality of life significantly. There are no clinical trials for buprenorphine patches specifically in arthritis but patients have been successfully transferred from weak oral opiates to transdermal buprenorphine patches in a variety of chronic pain syndromes. Both opiates are well-tolerated but the most common adverse events are similar to oral opiates including nausea, vomiting and constipation. Local adverse events, including pruritus, dermatitis and erythema, occur in about 1% of patients.

Many other drugs can improve pain in arthritis. Tricyclic antidepressants such as amitriptyline can be used to control pain and improve sleep. However, the evidence base is incomplete and patients may vary considerably in response; some clinicians use them extensively but others only rarely. Their beneficial effects on pain must be weighed against their side effects and the drowsiness they can cause, which may be worsened by other concomitant therapy. One important complication of opiates is an increased risk of falls.

5.2.3 Non steroidal anti-inflammatory drugs (NSAIDs)

This diverse group of drugs control inflammatory pain and some other symptoms of inflammation such as tenderness and stiffness though they have relatively limited impact on joint swelling or on systemic signs of inflammation such as an elevated ESR. NSAIDs inhibit cyclo-oxygenase (COX), which has a key role in prostaglandin synthesis. It occurs in two isoforms, COX-1 which is responsible for "housekeeping" prostaglandins involved in normal renal, gastric and vascular function, and COX-2 which is induced at sites of inflammation. The most common classification of NSAIDs differentiates drugs by their relative capacity to inhibit COX-1 versus COX-2. It was thought that COX-2 specific NSAIDs would have less effect on normal physiological function. However, NSAIDs may exert their effects through other mechanisms of action including uncoupling of oxidative phosphorylation, inhibition of lysosomal enzyme release and complement activation, antagonism of kinins and inhibition of free radicals.

There are a range of NSAIDs available with different dosing schedules. Commonly used conventional NSAIDs include ibuprofen, diclofenac and naproxen. Frequent dosing provides greater flexibility for individual patients, but also means taking more tablets at frequent intervals.

Once daily treatment is more convenient, but risks greater toxicity. Side effects are minimised by giving the lowest dose compatible with symptom relief. Systematic reviews have found no major differences in efficacy between the currently available NSAIDs, though there are differences in response of individuals and in adverse reactions.

Adverse effects are a major limiting factor using NSAIDs. Risks increase with age; therefore NSAIDs must be used carefully in the elderly. Minor adverse effects such as dyspepsia and headache are commonplace and rashes also occur. Renal, gastro-intestinal and cardiac side effects cause more problems. Central nervous system side effects, such as drowsiness and confusion, are often underestimated. Haematological side effects are unusual. NSAIDs can exacerbate pre-existing asthma. Gastrointestinal adverse events are a major concern, and these include serious problems such as ulceration, bleeding and perforation. Co medication with glucocorticoids or oral anticoagulants strongly increases this risk. The risks can be reduced by co-prescribing a proton pump inhibitor such as omeprazole.

Identifying the COX-II isoenzyme provided a new therapeutic target. The hope was to achieve similar anti-inflammatory action and pain relief to conventional NSAIDs, but without gastro-intestinal toxicity associated with COX-1 inhibition. Commonly used COX-II specific drugs include celecoxib and etoricoxib. Although several new COX-II specific drugs were developed, a number of them resulted in significant non-gastro-intestinal toxicities, particularly cardiac adverse effects, and several COX-II specific such as a rofecoxib and valdecoxib were subsequently withdrawn.

Coxibs are all equally effective in patient groups when compared with conventional NSAIDs. They have less gastro-intestinal toxicity and decrease the risk of gastric ulcers. However, their increased risk of cardiac adverse effects, particularly in patients with pre-existing cardiac disease and associated cardiac risk factors, limit their value. Other side effects are similar to conventional NSAIDs.

NSAIDs can be used topically as cream or gels; for example voltarol emulgel. These local NSAIDs are modestly effective and very safe. They are used mainly in osteoarthritis and soft tissue conditions rather than in rheumatoid arthritis. The use of combinations of low dose NSAIDs plus paracetamol (acetaminophen) appears to be as effective as, but safer than maximum dose NSAID.

5.2.4 Special situations

NSAIDs are relatively contraindicated in patients with pre-existing renal, hepatic or cardiac failure; other treatments are preferable. NSAIDs should be used cautiously or avoided in patients with asthma, because they can exacerbate bronchospasm. NSAIDs should be used with caution or best avoided in patients taking warfarin.

NSAIDs are not recommended during the first and third trimesters of pregnancy; in the first trimester they may be teratogenic and in the third trimester they may cause premature closure of the fetal ductus arteriosus and are linked with premature birth.

5.3 Disease-modifying anti-rheumatic drugs (DMARDs)

5.3.1 Available drugs and indications

DMARDs are a diverse group of drugs that both improve symptoms and also modify the course of the disease. This means that they reduce swelling of joints, improve general well being, decrease an elevated ESR and also slow or halt radiographic joint damage and reduce disability. Widely used DMARDs are listed in Table 5.2.

Methotrexate is the dominant 'anchor' drug for most patients, given to more than 80% of patients treated with DMARDs. Sulfasalazine, hydroxychloroquine, and leflunomide are also used commonly. Currently other DMARDs, including injectable gold, which was the first DMARD, are only rarely used.

Table 5.2 Main Disease-Modifying Anti-Rheumatic Drugs (DMARDs) in RA		
Frequently used	Typical dose regimen	Monitoring
Methotrexate	10–25 mg per week usually oral but can be given by sc injection	WCC, platelets and liver function tests every 4 weeks
Sulfasalazine	2 g per day	WCC, platelets and liver function tests every 4–12 weeks
Leflunomide	10–20 mg per day	BP, WCC, platelets and liver function tests every 4 weeks
Hydroxychloroquine	200–400 mg per day	Visual acuity and fundoscopy if using high dose
Occasionally used		
Azathioprine	2–2.5 mg/kg/day	WCC, platelets and liver function tests every 4 weeks
Ciclosporin	2.5–4 mg/kg/day	BP, WCC, platelets and liver function tests every 4 weeks
Injectable gold (sodium aurothio-malate)	50 mg per week reducing to 50 mg per month	WCC, platelets and uri-nalysis for protein as frequently as the injection

5.3.2 **Methotrexate**

Methotrexate is an anti-metabolite that inhibits folate metabolism, although it appears to act as an anti-inflammatory agent in the low doses (up to 25mg/week) used in arthritis. These low doses may have other effects, such as changing adenosine metabolism and accumulation in white cells. It is given weekly, usually orally, but it can also be given by subcutaneous or intramuscular injections to enhance absorption and reduce gastrointestinal side effects. Methotrexate is strongly bound to plasma proteins, and could be displaced by drugs like NSAIDs. However, this is not a problem in practice. Methotrexate is usually initiated orally at a dose of 7.5–15 mg/week. This is increased to a target dose of, on average, 15 mg-20 mg/week, though higher doses have been used. Lower doses are given if the drug is poorly tolerated. Methotrexate is given with low dose folic acid to reduce adverse reactions.

It is important to distinguish between weekly low-lose methotrexate used to treat RA, and high-dose methotrexate used to treat neoplastic disease. High-dose methotrexate may cause many side effects, leading to an image of methotrexate as a dangerous drug, while weekly low-dose methotrexate leads to few side effects in the majority of patients. Common gastrointestinal adverse effects often resolve with dose reduction or parenteral administration. Stomatitis is frequent. Alopecia causes concern in women but is usually mild and always reversible. Methotrexate may cause accelerated nodulosis, with small nodules on the fingers or elbows; this may respond to treatment with hydroxychloroquine. Infections, including opportunistic infections and herpes zoster sometimes occur.

Serious side effects include cytopenias, most commonly leucopenia, which responds to methotrexate withdrawal. Mild transaminase elevations are common, but serious hepatotoxicity, which can lead to fibrosis or frank cirrhosis, is rare. Methotrexate should be avoided in patients with risks of liver damage such as a high alcohol intake. A potentially lethal acute pneumonitis occurs rarely, and methotrexate should be stopped if patients develop respiratory symptoms such as a persisting dry cough.

Patients should be monitored prior to and during treatment with methotrexate. Conventionally full blood counts and liver function tests are undertaken every 1–3 months. A chest X-ray is taken at the beginning of treatment, so that any subsequent lung problems can be evaluated from a known baseline.

5.3.3 **Sulfasalazine**

Sulfasalazine combines an anti-inflammatory agent (5-aminosalicylic acid) with a sulfonamide antibiotic (sulfapyridine), which is thought to be the active component. There is extensive metabolism of sulfasalazine and its two constituents after the drug is ingested. Sulfasalazine is given orally with a target dose of 2–3 g daily. To minimise upper gastrointestinal side effects such as nausea, treatment is initiated at 500 mg daily rising slowly to 2 or 3 g per day. Sulfasalazine may cause a number of side effects in addition to gastrointestinal disturbances including rashes, reduced white cell counts and a rise in liver enzymes. It requires monitoring for blood and liver toxicity, particularly in the early stages. A particular concern is an unpredictable allergic reaction which may include neutropenia that can occur at any stage of treatment.

5.3.4 Hydroxychloroquine

Hydroxychloroquine is modestly effective in RA, especially in early disease. It is usually given at a dose of 400 mg/day. It is less effective than other DMARDs in most patients, but it is relatively safe and is actually used in up to 50% of patients. It is particularly valuable when taken in conjunction with methotrexate and sulfasalazine as triple combination therapy (see section 5.3.7). Adverse effects include rash, abdominal cramps and diarrhoea. Opinions vary on whether hydroxychloroquine (as opposed to chloroquine) causes retinopathy but the risk at prescribed doses is extremely low.

5.3.5 Leflunomide

Leflunomide was developed as an immunosuppressant for RA. It is a pyrimidine synthesis inhibitor with anti-proliferative activity. Leflunomide is a pro-drug with a half life of 2 weeks, which is converted in the gastrointestinal tract and plasma to its active metabolite.

The effective dose of leflunomide is 20 mg daily; some patients benefit from 10 mg daily. An initial loading dose (100 mg per day for 3 days) may result in more rapid response, but also results in more early side effects, especially gastro-intestinal reactions, and is not in widespread use.

Common adverse reactions include diarrhoea, nausea, reversible alopecia and rashes. Diarrhoea often leads to patients stopping treatment. Hypertension is seen some cases. There is also a small increased risk of infections, in common with other immunosuppressive drugs. Occasional patients develop low white cell counts or low platelet counts, and treatment should be stopped.

One particular concern is liver damage. Transient increases in liver enzymes are commonplace, and can usually be managed by careful observation. If the levels rise to more than three times the normal level, treatment should be stopped. A few patients have developed cirrhosis or liver failure. Patients receiving leflunomide need regular monitoring of liver function and blood counts. These are undertaken more frequently for the first 6 months and less often thereafter. Blood pressure should also be monitored since hypertension may occur as a side effect, and require treatment.

A washout procedure, using cholestyramine or activated powdered charcoal for 1–2 weeks, can be considered for overdose, severe side effects, after unintended conception, or as a planned procedure prior to an intentional pregnancy.

5.3.6 **Other DMARDs**

Azathioprine is used because of its immunosuppressive effects. It improves symptoms in some patients, but has less efficacy and more toxicity than other DMARDs in most patients. Haematological toxicity limits its value, but it is not contraindicated during pregnancy.

Ciclosporin is an immunosuppressive drug that improves symptoms and decreases erosive damage. Its adverse effects, particularly nephro-toxicity and hypertension, limit its long-term use. It may be useful to control flares over a few months.

Gold injection therapy may be as effective as methotrexate in many patients, but is frequently stopped because of adverse reactions, some of which can be serious. The use of gold has therefore markedly reduced in recent years. Gold is given as weekly injections of sodium aurothiomalate 50 mg intramuscularly and after up to 20 injections is decreased to 50 mg every month. It may cause proteinuria or rashes, which may persist long after treatment is stopped, as well as marrow failure, which may be a fatal outcome almost never seen with meth-otrexate or sulfasalazine. Careful monitoring of blood counts and urine is required.

5.3.7 **Combining DMARDS**

Despite conventional therapy with DMARDs many patients have an aggressive course with progressive joint destruction and marked disability developing over 5–10 years or longer. There is evidence that early therapy with DMARDs improves outcome and that two or more DMARDs used together are more effective than single DMARDs used sequentially. Combinations which include glucocorti-coid therapy have also been shown to be effective (see later section on glucocorticoids).

Effective combinations are summarized in Table 5.3. They include methotrexate with sulfasalazine and hydroxychloroquine, metho-rexate with ciclosporin; and methotrexate with leflunomide. Using two or more DMARDs at the same time may increase the chance of toxicity, and combinations must be used with careful monitoring.

Table 5.3 Main DMARD combinations

Combination	Comment
Methotrexate, Hydroxychloroquine, Sulfasalazine	Effective, safe and widely used
Methotrexate, Leflunomide	Effective, risks of liver toxicity
Methotrexate, Ciclosporin	Effective, risks of renal toxicity
Methotrexate, Gold	Limited evidence
Leflunomide, Sulfasalazine	Limited evidence
Leflunomide, Ciclosporin	Limited evidence

Figure 5.1 Benefits of early treatment with DMARDs in slowing radiographic damage

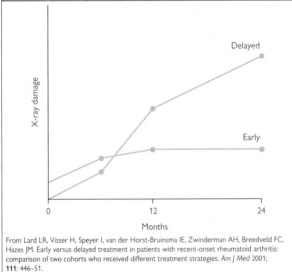

From Lard LR, Visser H, Speyer I, van der Horst-Bruinsma IE, Zwinderman AH, Breedveld FC, Hazes JM. Early versus delayed treatment in patients with recent-onset rheumatoid arthritis: comparison of two cohorts who received different treatment strategies. Am J Med 2001; **111**: 446–51.

5.3.8 Early treatment

There is a growing consensus that DMARDs should be used as early as possible. Observational studies show that patients with active RA in whom DMARDs are started early have better functional and radiological outcomes after 2–5 years (Figure 5.1). Randomized trials support these observational findings. Trials of early treatment with sulfasalazine and/ or hydroxychloroquine demonstrated reduced disease activity and radiographic damage.

5.3.9 Withdrawing DMARDs

When RA patients taking DMARDs achieve remission, stopping therapy increases the risk of a flare. On the other hand, many patients are reluctant to continue with potentially toxic drugs if they have been in remission for many years. The problem of stopping therapy in RA is similar to hypertension and diabetes (and all dysregulatory diseases) for which there is no 'cure', and where indefinite treatment is usually required. Withdrawal should be considered only in those patients who are in prolonged clinical and laboratory remission. All risks and potential benefits should be discussed in detail with the patient; as always, particularly the patient's in the absence of definitive data, opinion should be carefully considered.

5.3.10 Pregnancy

Many DMARDs including methotrexate and leflunomide are teratogenic and best avoided before and during pregnancy. Treatment should be stopped before attempting conception. The optimal gap differs between drugs: 3–6 months for methotrexate and 2 years for leflunomide (unless the latter is washed out using cholestyramine or activated charcoal – see section 5.3.3). By contrast, hydroxychloroquine, sulfasalazine, azathioprine, and ciclosporin have all been used safely in pregnancy.

5.4 Glucocorticoids

5.4.1 Available drugs

Glucocorticoids are injected locally into joints for active arthritis or into the soft tissues to deal with tenosynovitis and other local problems. They can also be given systemically either as one or more IM injections or orally at high or low dose. In all these settings they are effective in the short-term, less beneficial in the medium to long-term, and associated in the long-term with many significant adverse events in doses higher than 5 mg/day. It has proved challenging to balance their short term efficacy with their long term adverse effects.

5.4.2 Local

Injections of steroids, often in combination with a local anaesthetic, into joints, tendon sheaths and similar soft tissue sites is simple, safe and relatively effective in providing symptomatic relief. There is a limited formal evidence base because few trials have been undertaken. There are potential risks from sepsis and tendon rupture, but these are rare. Skin depigmentation may occur and is especially noticeable in patients with dark skin; they can reassured that it is usually localised, but may be permanent and accompanied by atrophy.

5.4.3 Systemic

Glucocorticoids are uniquely effective in RA. High doses are almost uniformly remittive, but result in unacceptable side effects. Brief pulses of high doses are much safer, but the true risk/benefit balance is not known. Recent trials have shown that low-to-intermediate dosing (3–15 mg/d prednisolone) added to conventional DMARDs is safe and results in better outcome, especially in terms of progression of damage in early patients. Combination of an oral pulse of glucocorticoid followed by a low dose, together with MTX and SSZ has been shown to be as effective as high-dose MTX and infliximab (a TNF inhibitor, see next chapter). Patients treated with this schedule showed an ongoing protection against damage progression compared to SSZ alone up to 5 years, even though treatment and disease activity were comparable and glucocorticoid were mostly discontinued after 6–12 months.

Nevertheless, there is an ongoing debate about the overall value of steroids. Many experts believe they are safe and beneficial when cautiously used in doses of 5mg per day or less and should be given to most patients at least as part of an induction regimen. Others feel that the benefits are modest yet their risks are substantial, and try to avoid steriods unless required for treatment of life-threatening disease.

5.4.4 Adverse events

The severity of side effects limits the value of steroid therapy in doses greater than 5 mg/day, particularly in the medium or long term. Steroids have many serious risks including osteoporosis, weight gain, hypertension, an increased risk of diabetes, infections and skin thinning; excessive dosage can lead to a Cushingoid appearance. Many of these effects are limited, if patients are given proper management. Patients should have bone protection if steroids are given for any length of time; this includes the use of calcium and vitamin D and bisphosphonates such as weekly alendronate or risedronate.

5.5 Patient information

Patients should be given both verbal and written information about the treatments they receive. These should outline the main effects, likely timeframe of improvements, the key adverse events and any significant risks. Many hospitals have developed local information sheets on the main DMARDs, and charitable organizations provide on-line information for patients; for example the Arthritis Research Campaign (http://www.arc.org.uk). Patients should also be reminded of the severe natural history of untreated RA, which can be similar to cancer and cardiovascular disease in terms of reducing life expectancy; the effects of the disease far outweigh the theoretical risks of the drugs.

Given the lack of knowledge about anti-rheumatic drugs by non-rheumatology health professionals, best practice is that patients can contact a rheumatology nurse or doctor if they have concerns about their therapy, for example through a help line (see Chapter 7).

Further reading

Choy EH, Smith C, Doré CJ, Scott DL. A meta-analysis of the efficacy and toxicity of combining disease-modifying anti-rheumatic drugs in rheumatoid arthritis based on patient withdrawal. *Rheumatology* 2005; **44**: 1414–21.

Donahue KE, Gartlehner G, Jonas DE, Lux LJ, Thieda P, Jonas BL, Hansen RA, Morgan LC, Lohr KN. Systematic review: comparative effectiveness and harms of disease-modifying medications for rheumatoid arthritis. *Ann Intern Med* 2008; **148**: 124–34.

Olsen NJ, Stein CM. New drugs for rheumatoid arthritis. *N Engl J Med* 2004; **350**: 2167–79.

Pincus T, Ferraccioli G, Sokka T, Larsen A, Rau R, Kushner I, Wolfe F. Evidence from clinical trials and long-term observational studies that disease-modifying anti-rheumatic drugs slow radiographic progression in rheumatoid arthritis: updating a 1983 review. *Rheumatology* 2002; **41**: 1346–56.

Quinn MA, Conaghan PG, Emery P. The therapeutic approach of early intervention for rheumatoid arthritis: what is the evidence? *Rheumatology* 2001; **40**: 1211–20.

Chapter 6

Biologic therapy

Peter Taylor

Key points

- Biologic therapies for RA are protein-based drugs which target specific components of the immune system known to be of pathogenic relevance
- Biologic therapeutics targeting tumor neurosis factor alpha (TNFα) have been successful in suppressing inflammation and markedly inhibiting the progression of structural damage; five anti-TNF agents are now available: adalimumab, certolizumab pegol, etanercept, golimumab, and infliximab
- Biological TNFα inhibitors have greatest efficacy for improvement in symptoms and signs and prevention of structural damage when used in combination with methotrexate
- Rituximab is a biologic agent that depletes B cells for use after failure of an anti-TNF biologic agent
- Abatacept, which targets the co-stimulatory pathway of inflammation, is approved for use in many countries (but not in the UK)
- Other biologic therapies directed against different immune targets have been licensed for use in RA or are in development but have not yet been approved by NICE
- Several new, non-biologic agent approaches to immuno-modulatory therapy for RA are also in development.

6.1 What is biologic therapy?

'Biologic' therapies are protein-based drugs derived from living organisms that are designed to either inhibit or augment a specific component of the immune system. Examples include antibodies directed against very specific molecular components of the immune response, for example, pro-inflammatory cytokines such as TNFα or interleukin (IL)-6. A potential advantage of a highly targeted therapeutic is the avoidance of toxic effects that a drug may have on molecular pathways other than their effects on the primary therapeutic target. Even so, where a biologic agent is directed against a single component of the immune system, mechanism-related toxicity may arise.

6.2 **The role of biologic targeted therapy and relationship with pathogenesis**

The primary cause of rheumatoid arthritis (RA) remains unknown. Nonetheless, advances in molecular technology have facilitated identification of numerous novel therapeutic targets, including cytokines, cell subsets, and co-stimulatory molecules, that contribute to the inflammatory and destructive components of rheumatoid arthritis. Concurrent advances in biotechnology have made it possible to produce abundant high-quality chimerized mouse-human or even completely human monoclonal antibodies with specificity for relevant disease molecules. Other approaches to blocking pro-inflammatory molecules include the use of naturally occurring soluble receptors or inhibitory proteins.

Biological therapies directed against several different molecular targets have so far been licensed in Europe and the USA for use in RA (Table 6.1).

These targets include the pro-inflammatory cytokines tumour necrosis factor α (TNFα) and interleukin-1 (IL-1), and interleukin-6 (IL-6); a subset of lymphocytes comprising B cells expressing the CD20 antigen; and the co-stimulatory signal provided by an interaction between members of the B-7 family (either CD80 or 86) on antigen-presenting cells and CD28 on T cells. Of these, only three TNFα inhibitors and the B cell depleting agent rituximab are approved in the UK by the National Institute for Health and Clinical Excellence as being cost effective.

Many other biologic therapies are in development for RA and have yet to be licensed for use (Table 6.1). These include further TNF inhibitors, a second generation of B cell depleting agents, other approaches targeting B cells, antibodies directed against the pro-inflammatory cytokine interleukin-6 (IL-6) and antibodies to Receptor Activator for Nuclear Factor κ B Ligand (RANKL), a molecule important to bone metabolism that promotes osteoclast activation and bone resorption.

6.2.1 TNFα inhibitors

Five biologic TNF inhibitors are currently available for clinical practice (Figure 6.1). These are infliximab, a chimeric monoclonal anti-TNFα antibody comprising a human IgG-1κ antibody with a mouse variable region fragment of high affinity and neutralizing capacity; adalimumab, a monoclonal human antibody produced by phage display; and etanercept, an engineered p75 TNF receptor dimer with a fully human amino acid sequence linked to the Fc portion of human IgG1. Certolizumab pegol is a PEGylated anti-TNF agent with a high affinity for human TNF-alpha, and golimumab which has a similar mechanism of action to infliximab, but differs by being fully humanized and is given as a subcutaneous injection. The monoclonal antibodies have specificity for TNFα. In contrast, the fusion protein etanercept acts as a competitive inhibitor of TNFA

Molecular target	Biologic therapy	Licensed for RA treatment in the UK	Approved by NICE in England and Wales	Licensed for use in USA	Licensed for use in Europe
TNFα	Infliximab	Yes	Yes	Yes	Yes
TNFα	Adalimumab	Yes	Yes	Yes	Yes
TNFα/β	Etanercept	Yes	Yes	Yes	Yes
TNFα	Golimumab	Yes	Being considered	Yes	Yes
TNFα	Certolizumab Pegol	Yes	Being considered	Yes	Yes
IL-1	Anakinra (IL-1 receptor antagonist)	Yes	No	Yes	Yes
IL-6 Receptor	Tocilizumab	Yes	No	Yes	Yes
B cells expressing CD20	Rituximab	Yes	Yes (in anti-TNF failures)	Yes	Yes
B cells expressing CD20	Ocrelizumab	In development		In development	In development
B cells expressing CD20	Ofatumumab	In development		In development	In development
B7/CD28 co-stimulation pathway	Abatacept	Yes	No	Yes	Yes
RANK ligand	Denosumab	In development		In development	In development
IL-23	Apilimod	In development		In development	In development
IL-17		In development		In development	In development

Table 6.1 Biologic therapies

and can also bind lymphotoxin (TNFB). A number of mechanisms of action for TNF inhibitors relevant to the pathogenesis of RA are listed in Box 6.1.

6.2.2 B cell targeting

Rituximab, a B cell depleting monoclonal anti-CD20 antibody, is the first biologic agent targeting B cells to be approved in the USA and Europe for the treatment of active RA in anti-TNF non-responders. The role of B cells in the pathogenesis of RA is not fully understood. Nonetheless, there are a number of known B cell functions of likely relevance, including their role in antigen presentation, secretion of pro-inflammatory cytokines, production of rheumatoid factor and thus their role in immune complex formation, and co-stimulation of T cells. Of note, immune complexes are one trigger to production of

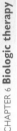

> **Figure 6.1 UK-licensed biologic inhibitors of TNFα for the treatment of RA.**

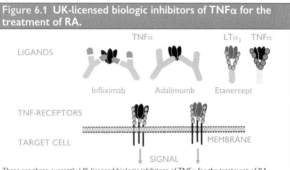

There are three currently UK-licensed biologic inhibitors of TNFα for the treatment of RA. Infliximab is a chimaeric monoclonal antibody that includes murine amino-acid sequences in the variable region of the immunoglobulin. Adalimumab is a monoclonal antibody with a fully human amino-acid sequence and etanercept is a fusion protein comprising an engineered p75 TNF receptor dimer with a fully human amino acid sequence linked to the Fc portion of human IgG1.

Box 6.1 Mechanisms of action of TNFα inhibitors

- De-activation of the pro-inflammatory cytokine cascade at the site of inflammation
- Reduction in mediators of joint destruction
- Diminished recruitment of inflammatory cells from the blood to the rheumatoid joint
- Diminished synovial vascularity.

TNF and other pro-inflammatory cytokines. B cells are also implicated in the process of ectopic lymphoid organogenesis in the rheumatoid synovium. Clinical studies of rituximab demonstrate that it can be effective in up to 50% of patients who fail to respond to TNF inhibitors.

6.2.3 Inhibition of co-stimulatory molecules

Abatacept, which interferes with co-stimulatory molecule signalling has been shown to be an effective treatment for RA licensed for use in the USA and some European countries. It selectively modulates CD80 or CD86 on the surface of antigen presenting cells. These molecules normally bind to CD28 on lymphocytes as part of the second signal of T cell activation (see chapter 2). The natural inhibitor of this interaction is cytotoxic T lymphocyte antigen 4 (CTLA4) and abatacept is a fusion protein containing CTLA4 and an Fc portion of Ig. There have been a number of promising studies demonstrating good control of synovitis.

6.3 Guidelines on the use of TNF inhibitors

The high production costs and overall expense of biologic agents render it is necessary to operate within the health economic constraints of any given healthcare system. In practice, this may mean that certain therapies are available only when used within a setting of nationally agreed guidelines. In the UK, such guidelines are set by the National Institute for Health and Clinical Excellence (NICE). Extracts from the guidance for use of the anti-TNF biologics infliximab, etanercept and adalimumab and the B cell depleting biologic rituximab are given in Box 6.2 and 6.3 respectively.

> **Box 6.2 Specific aspects of patient care covered by NICE guidance for the tumour necrosis factor alpha (TNFα) inhibitors adalimumab, etanercept and infliximab**
>
> - The tumour necrosis factor alpha (TNFα) inhibitors adalimumab, etanercept, and infliximab are recommended as options for the treatment of adults who have both of the following characteristics:
>   - Active rheumatoid arthritis as measured by disease activity score (DAS28) greater than 5.1 confirmed on at least two occasions, 1 month apart
>   - Have undergone trials of two disease-modifying anti-rheumatic drugs (DMARDs), including methotrexate (unless contraindicated). A trial of a DMARD is defined as being normally of 6 months, with 2 months at standard dose, unless significant toxicity has limited the dose or duration of treatment
> - TNFα inhibitors should normally be used in combination with methotrexate. Where a patient is intolerant of methotrexate or where methotrexate treatment is considered to be inappropriate, adalimumab or etanercept may be given as monotherapy
> - Treatment with TNFα inhibitors should be continued beyond 6 months only if there is an adequate response at 6 months following initiation of therapy. An adequate response is defined as an improvement in DAS28 of 1.2 units or more
> - After initial response, treatment should be monitored no less frequently than 6-monthly intervals with assessment of DAS28. Treatment should be withdrawn if an adequate response is not maintained
> - An alternative TNFα inhibitor may be considered for patients in whom treatment is withdrawn due to an adverse event before the initial 6-month assessment of efficacy, provided the risks and benefits have been fully discussed with the patient and documented
> - Use of the TNFα inhibitors for the treatment of severe, active and progressive rheumatoid arthritis in adults not previously treated with methotrexate or other DMARDs is not recommended
> - Initiation of TNFα inhibitors and follow-up of treatment response and adverse events should be undertaken only by a specialist rheumatological team with experience in the use of these agents.

Box 6.3 Specific aspects of patient care covered by NICE guidance for rituximab

- Rituximab in combination with methotrexate is recommended as an option for the treatment of adults with severe active rheumatoid arthritis who have had an inadequate response to or intolerance of other disease-modifying anti-rheumatic drugs (DMARDs), including treatment with at least one tumour necrosis factor α (TNFα) inhibitor therapy.
- Treatment with rituximab plus methotrexate should be continued only if there is an adequate response following initiation of therapy. An adequate response is defined as an improvement in disease activity score (DAS28) of 1.2 units or more.
- Repeat courses of treatment with rituximab plus methotrexate should be given no more frequently than every 6 months.
- Treatment with rituximab plus methotrexate should be initiated, supervised and treatment response assessed by specialist physicians experienced in the diagnosis and treatment of rheumatoid arthritis.

6.4 What is the long-term evidence for benefit or harm?

Data from numerous clinical trials with the anti-TNF agents infliximab, etanercept, and adalimumab have confirmed the validity of TNFα as a therapeutic target in rheumatoid arthritis. Similar data are emerging for the newer generation of biologic TNF inhibitors including golimumab and certolizumab pegol. The major clinical benefits reported in clinical trials are listed in Box 6.4. Certolizumab pegol and golimumab, are licensed in the UK, have been approved in the USA, and have gained positive opinion from the EMEA Committee for Medicinal Products for Human Use (CHMP).

The effectiveness of a treatment in improving the symptoms and signs of RA can be assessed in the context of clinical trials using validated tools such as DAS28 or the American College of Rheumatology (ACR) response (see Chapter 4). Studies of TNFα inhibitor treatment have been performed in patients with RA who have failed to respond adequately to multiple DMARD therapies, in whom there is active disease despite ongoing methotrexate therapy. Between 50 and 70% of patients are reported to achieve an ACR 20 response level at six months, as compared to between 20–30% of patients continued on methotrexate alone. At the more stringent ACR 50 response level, the difference between the proportion of

Box 6.4 Clinical benefits of TNF blockade

- Reduction of symptoms, including pain, stiffness, and lethargy
- Reduction in signs of active disease, including joint swelling and tenderness
- Reduction in cartilage and bone damage
- Remission induction
- Preservation and improvement of functional status.

Box 6.5 Key safety considerations for biologic TNFα antagonists

- Infection, both common and opportunistic
- Cytopaenias
- Demyelinating disease
- Lupus-like syndromes
- Congestive heart failure
- Malignancies, particularly lymphomas.

patients with established disease responding on methotrexate alone and those responding on the combination of methotrexate and a TNFα inhibitor is approximately 20–40% at one year. At the ACR 70 response level, approximately 15% of patients will respond compared to only 1% of patients on conventional DMARDs.

TNFα blockade significantly inhibits radiographic damage to joints, as shown by a study demonstrating dose-dependent reductions in serum concentrations of mediators of cartilage degradation, and confirmed in longer term studies looking at reduced progression of joint space narrowing and erosions in patients treated with TNFα blockade plus methotrexate. Subsequent studies showed that therapy with an anti-TNF biologic agent and methotrexate halts progression of joint damage in RA not only in patients with limited radiographic destruction at baseline, but also in some (not all) with extensive damage.

There are data for all three currently available anti-TNF inhibitors to show that repeated therapy over time, in particular when an anti-TNF agent is combined with methotrexate, leads to significant improvement in physical function and quality of life.

For biologic therapies directed against TNFα, the key safety considerations are listed in Box 6.5.

Biological therapies targeting TNFα have greatest efficacy for improvement in symptoms and signs and prevention of structural damage when used in combination with methotrexate.

6.5 **Combination of biologic agent with DMARD**

The effects of TNFα blockade, with or without concomitant methotrexate therapy, have been compared with methotrexate alone in the early phase of rheumatoid arthritis, i.e. in patients not previously exposed to MTX. The findings of the studies indicate that biological therapies targeting TNFα have greatest efficacy for improvement in symptoms and signs of disease, remission induction, as well as prevention of structural damage, when used in combination with methotrexate. Furthermore, this apparent synergy can be achieved with modest methotrexate doses. Clinical experience in the use of anti-TNFα drugs confirms these findings in most patients.

6.6 **Beyond biologics: small molecules and stem-cell transplantation**

Despite the unprecedented clinical and commercial successes of biologic agents for the treatment of RA, particularly TNFα inhibitors used together with methotrexate, there are many compelling reasons to seek to improve on the outcomes achievable with currently available agents. One reason is that a minority of patients remain refractory to currently available biologic agent treatments. There is thus considerable interest in the development of new, less expensive, orally active, synthetic agents including those that inhibit bioactivity of TNFα and/or IL-1. Although a number of new "small molecule" approaches have been tested, several have not yet progressed to the clinic because of a disappointing magnitude of efficacy or unacceptable high toxicity. Examples include several inhibitors of the inflammatory molecule p38 MAP kinase, designed to block signaling in the p38 pathway and thus the post-transcriptional stabilization of mRNAs for the major inflammatory cytokines TNFα and IL-1, as well as other proteins such as cyclooxygenase-2. Other molecular targets of interest include Janus kinase 3 (JAK-3), a key component in the signal transduction cascade of numerous growth factors that is activated by multiple cytokines, and Spleen tyrosine kinase (Syk), a critical component in immune-complex-mediated signal transduction.

Since 1996, approximately 1,000 patients have received an autologous hematopoietic stem cell transplant as treatment for a severe autoimmune disease. The initially high treatment-related mortality has reduced significantly in the later years. However, although there are case reports of long-lasting remissions, most RA patients show only transient responses in disease activity, functional ability, quality of life and rate of joint destruction, although the disease may be more amenable to anti-rheumatic medication post-transplantation. In recent years there has been a growing interest in the role and potential therapeutic application of mesenchymal stem cells in the immunomodulation of autoimmune disease, as in the early experience with acute-graft-versus host disease.

Further reading

Breedveld FC, Weisman MH, Kavanaugh AF et al. The PREMIER study: A multicenter, randomized, double-blind clinical trial of combination therapy with adalimumab plus methotrexate versus methotrexate alone or adalimumab alone in patients with early, aggressive rheumatoid arthritis who had not had previous methotrexate treatment. *Arthritis Rheum* 2006; **54**: 26–37.

Cohen SB, Emery P, Greenwald MW et al. Rituximab for rheumatoid arthritis refractory to anti-tumor necrosis factor therapy: Results of a multicenter, randomized, double-blind, placebo-controlled, phase III trial evaluating primary efficacy and safety at twenty-four weeks. *Arthritis Rheum* 2006; **54**: 2793–2806.

Edwards JC, Szczepanski L, Szechinski J et al. Efficacy of B-cell-targeted therapy with rituximab in patients with rheumatoid arthritis. *N Engl J Med* 2004; **350**: 2572–81.

Emery P, Fleischmann R, Filipowicz-Sosnowska A et al. for The efficacy and safety of rituximab in patients with active rheumatoid arthritis despite methotrexate treatment. Results of a phase IIB randomized, double-blind, placebo-controlled, dose-ranging study. *Arthritis Rheum* 2006; **54**: 1390–1400.

Klareskog L, van der Heijde D, de Jager JP et al. Therapeutic effect of the combination of etanercept and methotrexate compared with each treatment alone in patients with rheumatoid arthritis: double-blind randomised controlled trial. *Lancet* 2004; **363**: 675–81.

Lipsky PE, van der Heijde DM, St Clair EW et al. Infliximab and methotrexate in the treatment of rheumatoid arthritis. Anti-Tumor Necrosis Factor Trial in Rheumatoid Arthritis with Concomitant Therapy Study Group. *N Engl J Med* 2000; **343**: 1594–1602.

Passweg J, Tyndall A. Autologous stem cell transplantation in autoimmune diseases. *Semin Hematol* 2007; **44**: 278–85.

Taylor PC. Rheumatoid Arthritis in practice. Royal Society of Medicine Press Ltd; 1st edn, 2006.

Voulgari PV. Emerging drugs for rheumatoid arthritis. *Expert Opinion on Emerging Drugs* 2008; **13**: 175–96.

Chapter 7

Multidisciplinary team management

Sheena Hennell, Zoe Stableford, Jane Flynn and Raashid Luqmani

Key points

- Patients with rheumatoid arthritis should be managed by a multi-disciplinary team, including the use of advice/help-lines for all patients and annual review for monitoring patients with established arthritis
- Exercise has physical and psychological benefits in RA; it improves function and reduces bone loss, but high impact exercise should be avoided in patients with advanced structural damage
- Physiotherapy and occupational therapy intervention can ameliorate or prevent problems with activities of daily living or employment
- A hand assessment is useful to ensure that the patient is able to undertake routine nail care
- Advice and education on good foot hygiene, well fitting footwear and self assessment are important in order to prevent ulceration and opportunistic infections
- The use of foot orthoses is common practice to reduce pain but unproven for prevention or lessening of deformity or preservation of function
- Cigarette smoking is associated with more radiographic progression and cardiovascular disease in RA.

In many countries it is common practice for patients with RA to be managed by a multidisciplinary team. By contrast, in the US, reimbursement patterns leave very few allied health professionals as specialists in rheumatology. Nevertheless, patients with rheumatoid arthritis may benefit from input from multi-disciplinary team care which includes many health professionals beyond physicians. Many of the measures proposed are supported by common sense but without evidence from randomized controlled trials or observational studies. Box 7.1 shows typical members of a team for patients

67

> ## Box 7.1 Typical membership of a multidisciplinary team for managing RA
>
> - Rheumatologist
> - Rheumatology practitioner/specialist nurse
> - Physiotherapist
> - Occupational therapist
> - Podiatrist
> - Orthotist
> - Orthopaedic surgeon
> - Psychologist
> - Dietician
> - Pharmacist
> - Social worker
> - Disability employment adviser

with RA. The composition of teams varies in different hospitals. Patients may achieve better outcomes if they are managed by specialist teams compared to the care that can be achieved by single handed practitioners. Team interventions can help patients to reduce the impact of arthritis on the individual, family and society. For some patients, it can be difficult to come to terms with having an incurable, chronic, disabling condition, and team members can offer support to enable patients to engage effectively in physiotherapy programmes and to benefit from occupational therapy advice for maintaining long-term function.

7.1 Patient education and support

In the UK (and other countries), rheumatology practitioners can provide patients with support by direct face to face meetings to discuss practical issues and education about the disease and its treatment, so that they can become active in managing some aspects of their own condition. In some other countries these tasks are performed by a variety of team members. A supportive relationship between the health care professional and patient can enhance self-esteem through coordinated care in order to develop coping strategies and support patient self-efficacy.

There are a number of local and national patient self help support groups, including voluntary organizations. They can provide information and support. In the UK, the National Rheumatoid Arthritis Society (NRAS) network provides support for patients with RA by way of introductions to other patients and carers. In Europe the European Arthritis Patient Organization provides excellent links to many national organizations in individual countries. In the United States of America, the American Arthritis Foundation provides similar support.

Patient education has become an important component of traditional management, providing strategies and tools which support patients in

> ### Box 7.2 Topics covered in a typical education programme for patients with RA
>
> - Disease process, progression and medical management
> - Drug information and monitoring
> - Social, psychological and emotional impact of the disease
> - Diet and nutrition
> - Accessing services/helpline
> - Exercise, joint protection, relaxation
> - Pain relief
> - Complementary therapies
> - Coping, goal setting
> - Self efficacy, self esteem, self management

making daily decisions in order to cope with rheumatoid arthritis and its treatment. Education includes written information, interactive programmes for groups of patients, as well as individual, one-to-one teaching.

The main aim is to provide education which is tailored to individual need or beliefs. The topics usually addressed in patient education programmes are outlined in Box 7.2.

Although patient education improves knowledge and behaviour, the effects are often only short term. However, patients find the information useful; developing their skills and knowledge can help to improve quality of life through self management and coping. Refreshers and updates from time to time are also useful.

7.2 The rheumatology nurse specialist/ rheumatology practitioner

Supporting patients and providing education and information within nurse led clinics or defined education sessions, has generally been the primary function of the nurse specialist/practitioner in the UK. However specialist nurses and other allied health professionals are now becoming increasingly autonomous, performing musculoskeletal assessments, undertaking joint injections, ordering investigations, interpreting results, making clinical decisions and prescribing.

7.3 Nurse or practitioner-led clinics

The nurse specialist/practitioner reviews a patient's disease activity. This includes the use of the disease activity score (DAS 28) to assess for tender and swollen joints (see Chapter 4). The nurse specialist/practitioner examines the patient's upper limb joints and knees and records the number of tender and swollen joints, the ESR and global health visual analogue score. Nurse specialist/practitioners use locally agreed protocols to facilitate treatment changes or titration of treatment including Disease-Modifying Anti-Rheumatic Drugs (DMARDs) and Biologics for patients, based on the severity of the patient's DAS 28 score – the higher the score the more likely that treatment will be escalated or changed. Patients are given the opportunity to discuss any concerns and ask questions and given information. The aim is to improve understanding, awareness of drug therapy side effects and promote concordance with treatment.

Assessment and nurse specialist/practitioner review also includes the Health Assessment Questionnaire (HAQ) to assess physical activity and the Hospital Anxiety and Depression Scale (HAD) to assess mood. Referral to physiotherapy and occupational therapy may be indicated if function is affected. Patients with depressed mood may benefit from psychological support provided by nurse specialists/practitioners and additional anti-depressant medication, if necessary.

7.4 Annual review

A comprehensive annual review offers a synthesis of patient self-management, primary care and hospital based care. It is useful for all patients, but possibly even more so for patients whose disease appears to be well controlled, and has remained quiescent for some time, typically 1 or 2 years from presentation. Elements that are considered to be important in the annual review are shown in Box 7.3.

An annual review could be undertaken in different health care settings but in many countries, hospital based rheumatology departments are most able to co-ordinate the process in partnership with general practitioners and patients. The core measurements and overall responsibility for different aspects of care should be agreed with each patient.

7.5 Rheumatology advice/help-line

In the UK, rheumatology healthcare professionals provide and operate an advice/help-line for patients, GPs and other health care professionals. This provides convenient and often immediate access to

Box 7.3 Typical elements of a comprehensive annual review

- Disease status, damage and patient function.
- Screening for co-morbidity
- Medications and adverse effects
- Educational needs
- Psychosocial issues
- Fatigue.
- Referral to other services in a multidisciplinary team or other related specialists.

accurate and reliable information. Patients may contact the helpline if they require advice on coping with flare, medication, general advice or information. Several studies report high levels of patient satisfaction for patients using the advice/help-line. Details of any treatment change are recorded in the patient's hospital notes and a letter is sent to the GP. If patients require an urgent review, urgent appointments at the nurse/practitioner-led clinic are available in most departments. GPs or practice nurses may also contact the help-line for advice and information, for monitoring problems or if urgent review is required.

7.6 Physiotherapy in rheumatoid arthritis

7.6.1 Exercise

Exercise provides physical and psychological benefits to patients by improving conditioning, self-efficacy and sense of well-being. By contrast, low levels of physical activity are associated with an increase in self reported stress. Regular exercise allows patients to take a more active role in the management their own disease. Many patients with early rheumatoid arthritis are mistakenly worried that exercise might make their condition worse, whereas in fact the opposite is true. There are 3 types of exercise which are helpful in the management of early RA (Table 7.1).

In elderly patients the use of progressive resistance training increases muscle strength and has a positive effect on function, although the effects on disability remain unclear. Patients with RA can undertake dynamic (aerobic) exercise without any adverse effects on their arthritis at least in the short term. Aerobic exercise is beneficial in terms of muscle strength, aerobic capacity, exercise tolerance and function. Excessive exercise is defined by the development of post-exercise fatigue lasting over an hour, increased joint swelling and pain.

Hydrotherapy is commonly practiced and can produce physiological, clinical and psychological benefits to patients, but there is a lack of well conducted studies.

Exercise is also effective in established rheumatoid arthritis. It improves function and reduces bone loss. The type of exercise and method of delivery that is most effective and cost-effective will vary considerably among individual patients. It is useful to assess patients for suitability for individual prescribed exercise so that tailor made exercise programmes can be developed.

Table 7.1 Exercises useful in management of early rheumatoid arthritis	
Range of movement exercises	Exercises through the current range of movement can maintain movement in joints and relieve stiffness. End of range non ballistic stretches may reduce development of contractures.
Strengthening exercises	Includes low resistance weight training to maintain muscle strength.
Aerobic endurance exercise	Includes cycling, swimming, and running which can improve cardiovascular fitness, help control weight, and improve overall function.

It is important to establish the factors that get and keep people exercising in order to derive long term benefit. Knowledge alone does not achieve this, but education linked to exercise with regular reinforcement by health professionals may be more effective. It is useful to explore the patient's attitudes toward physical activity in order to implement a healthy lifestyle which can encompass not only exercise, but also addresses diet, absence of cigarette smoking and limited alcohol consumption, all of which are important aspects of the care of patients with RA.

7.7 Smoking cessation

7.7.1 Association between smoking and RA

Comorbidity is important in the morbidity and mortality of RA. Cigarette smoking may have an adverse effect on radiographic progression (see chapter 1), and increases the risk of cardiovascular complications (see chapter 8) such as myocardial infarction; therefore it is appropriate to reduce risks wherever possible.

7.7.2 Interventions

All patients who smoke should be advised to quit. Individuals need to be willing to give up. Brief interventions of 5–10 minutes with a health care professional can provide opportunistic advice, discussion, negotiation or encouragement to quit. However, only a modest effect on smoking behaviour is reported; 2–3% of patients spontaneously give up and a further 1–3% stop smoking as a result of the intervention.

Health care professionals are encouraged to provide simple advice for quitting and offer pharmacotherapy and/or behavioural support. Provision of self-help material can assist patients who wish to quit; in the UK referral to NHS stop smoking services can ensure continuing support.

7.8 Intervention with heat, cold and physical measures

Heat and cold applications may relieve pain, stiffness, muscle spasm and swelling in some patients with rheumatoid arthritis. Heat is more effective in reducing stiffness, whilst cold is more useful for pain relief, especially in actively inflamed joints, although this varies from patient to patient. Paraffin wax baths can be used in combination with exercises to provide short-term relief for active hand arthritis, but are not commonly used. The main purpose of these interventions is to reduce pain so that the patient can participate in daily activities and therapeutic exercise.

The use of acupuncture-like transcutaneous electrical nerve stimulation (TENS) can reduce pain and improve strength, although some studies show that conventional TENS is no better than placebo (Figure 7.1 shows a TENS machine).

7.9 Occupational therapy

Occupational therapy interventions for patients with RA are listed in Table 7.2.

Figure 7.1 TENS machine

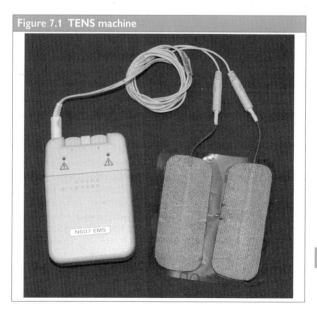

Table 7.2 Occupational therapy interventions in RA. Many interventions are common practice, but there is a lack of research to establish an evidence base

Therapy/Assessment	Purpose
Comprehensive therapy assessment	General approach encompassing all aspects of function to enable a treatment plan to be made
Environmental and home assessment	Evaluates areas for improvement
Training of skills	To improve ability to perform useful functions in those 60% of patients who have functional difficulties in the early course of their disease
Joint protection	Advice on avoiding inappropriate joint movements and improving efficiency
Energy conservation	Pacing, aimed at relieving fatigue which is very common in RA
Task modification	To enable the patient to continue performing appropriate tasks
Problem-solving exercises	Improve mobility, functioning and safety
Counselling	Adjusting expectation
Assistive devices	Particularly important for enhancing hand function e.g. use of jar openers, kettle tippers or tap turners
Resting splints	Resting splints decrease pain

During the course of RA patients can develop difficulties with mobility and function and commonly experience psychosocial problems. Pain, deformity, low energy and mood inhibit independent function. In established RA, most patients have difficulty with leisure activities and simple household activities. After 20 years of RA, most patients historically were moderately or severely disabled, although that appears to be changing at this time.

We advocate a structured approach towards rehabilitation management, and a key component is active participation of the patient. Hand function should be maintained and improved using a combination of hand exercises and appropriate devices to improve efficiency. Commonly affected activities include household tasks, leisure, work and parent and family roles. If patients have limitations to their leisure activities, this has an inevitable negative effect on their self esteem and their psychological status. We need to help patients to engage in these pursuits or alternative activities. It is important to help patients to regain functional independence through changing the way they perform tasks, as well as the use of assistive devices.

7.10 **Work disability rehabilitation**

Many people with rheumatoid arthritis experience limitations to their capacity to work; many cannot work or they can only work intermittently; other patients are at work but their performance is affected by their disease. If patients are working at the onset of disease, there is a one in three chance of becoming work disabled within five years, especially if they have poor levels of function (as measured using the HAQ see Chapter 4) and the job involves manual work. Other factors contributing to their ability to work include fatigue, lack of support, lack of autonomy and lack of participation in decision making. It may be useful for patients who are in employment to be reviewed regularly by an occupational therapist or rehabilitation counsellor in order to identify these risk factors so that support and advice could be offered. Disability Employment Advisors can provide financial and practical assistance. Occupational therapists and physiotherapists can be invaluable in helping patients to remain in work and improve their performance at work (see Box 7.4).

Work rehabilitation programmes can help patients to get back to work. Although vocational rehabilitation has been shown to reduce levels of fatigue and improve mental health, its impact on job retention is uncertain.

7.11 **Joint protection and assisted devices**

The use of assistive devices (see Figure 7.2) is more common in patients with established disease compared to early disease and can be invaluable in helping patients with eating, cooking and toileting. Every patient (and indeed non-patient) can benefit from some devices such as a jar opener. However we should remember that even though about half of all patients with RA own a walking aid, only two thirds of these patients actually use them.

A range of finger orthoses are available to correct deformities such as MCP joint ulnar drift, swan neck and boutonniere deformities and to improve hand function, but evidence for their effectiveness is limited. We suggest use of such appliances only when deformity is sufficiently reducible in order to improve hand function for the duration of a particular activity.

7.12 **Fatigue**

Fatigue, affects the quality of life of patients with rheumatoid arthritis and is an ongoing problem from the onset of disease. Reduction in activity and function over time is due to a variety of factors including muscle weakness, fatigue, attitude and motivation. When patients

- Work-based assessments
- Recommendations to modify work environment
- Provide appropriate assistive equipment
- Training in task modification
- Improved ergonomics
- Coping strategies
- Liaison with employers

Figure 7.2 Assistive devices to improve activity in RA

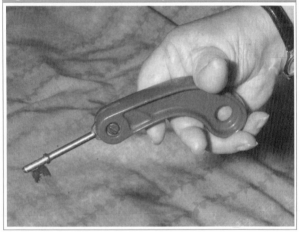

reduce their amount of physical activity because of fatigue it has a negative effect on their psychological well-being. Physical fatigue can be reduced by exercise and energy conservation techniques, for example pacing activities or simplifying tasks.

7.13 Orthotics and podiatry

7.13.1 Nail and skin problems in the foot

Nail problems are quite common in patients with RA. The most common problems relate to the inability to cut nails properly. This can cause in-growing toenails and increase the risk of infection. Long term immunosuppression as a result of RA and/or its treatment increases the risk of fungal infection of the skin and nails. Prompt treatment of these opportunistic infections is important to reduce risk of further tissue damage. Education should emphasize how self care is vital to optimum foot health.

Common skin conditions include callus formation over prominent metatarsal heads and retracted toes, due to ill fitting footwear. Callus should be reduced regularly if the area is painful or there is a risk of tissue breakdown. Emollients help maintain skin flexibility and should be used daily. The application of cream also encourages self inspection of feet to prompt early action and reduce the risk of further problems.

7.13.2 Prevention and treatment of the rheumatoid foot

A podiatrist offers routine nail care and callus reduction; nail surgery may be necessary in problematic nail conditions. Insoles or orthoses are used to accommodate or correct foot deformities. Patients should be assessed by a podiatrist early in their disease course to provide individual preventative advice and insoles if appropriate. The most common foot complaints are related to altered foot function and extra-articular features such as nodules, neuropathy and vasculitis. In patients with RA, the foot develops structural changes which affect normal function which in turn affects gait, mobility and impacts on quality of life.

Preventative and pain relief treatment include callus debridement, use of insoles or orthoses, surgical shoes and discussion on foot surgery. Patients can develop foot ulceration which is usually multi-factorial; a shared care approach between physicians, tissue viability nurses, district nurses and podiatry is recommended.

7.13.3 The role of insoles, shoes and podiatric surgery

Insoles, shoes or podiatric surgery should be used to achieve pain relief, prevent or correct deformity, preserve and restore function. Orthoses act functionally to prevent further deformity and increase function and mobility or accommodate the deformity to promote comfort when walking. Therefore, it is important to assess the movement of the foot and use the most appropriate device for the stage of disease. Foot orthoses can be used to stabilize the joint, for joint protection, for pain relief, to improve function, reduce inflammation or to rest joints or soft tissues.

When assessing the patients' own footwear, it is important to ensure that there is adequate width and room in the toe box. If deformity is present, such as hallux abducto valgus and retracted digits, the foot does not conform to retail measurements, and therefore patients may require assessment for surgical shoes. The assessment should be undertaken by an orthotist, including consideration for an orthotic device. Because RA is more common in women, it is important to incorporate the patient's views according to the choice of footwear. This will help to ensure the shoes are actually worn and also reduce the risk of skin trauma from wearing inappropriate shoes.

There has been very little research into the role of podiatric surgery in RA. Patients with RA have a high incidence of infection, therefore, wounds should be closely monitored post operatively and appropriate antibiotics used where indicated. In patients treated with TNFα inhibitors, there is no definitive guidance on stopping treatment before an elective procedure but with continuation of DMARDs there seems to be no additional risk of infection.

Suggested reading

Barouk LS, Barouk P. (2007) Joint-preserving surgery in rheumatoid forefoot: preliminary study with more-than-two-year follow-up. *Foot Ankle Clin.* 2007; **12**: 435–54, vi.

Firth J, Hale C, Helliwell P, Hill J, Nelson EA.(2008) The prevalence of foot ulceration in patients with rheumatoid arthritis. *Arthritis Rheum.* 2008 Feb **59**: 200–5.

Helliwell P, Woodburn J, Redmond A, Turner D, Davys H. (2007) *The Foot and Ankle in Rheumatoid Arthritis A Comprehensive Guide.* Churchill Livingstone Elsevier.

Linton SM and Meadows AJ (2001) Patients perception of a rheumatology helpline. *Rheumatology*: **40**: 1071–2.

Schreiber L and Colley M (2004). Patient education. *Best Pract Res Clin Rheumatol.* **18**: 465–7.

Masdottir B, Jonsson T, Manfredsdottir V, Vikingsson A, Brekkan A, Valdimarsson H Smoking, rheumatoid factor isotypes and severity of rheumatoid arthritis. *Rheumatology* (Oxford) 2000, **39**: 1202–5.

NICE Brief interventions and referral for smoking cessation in primary care and other settings (2006). NICE.

Saag, K.G., Cerhan, J.R., Kolluri, S. et al. (1997) Cigarette smoking and rheumatoid arthritis severity. *Annals of the Rheumatic Diseases* **56**(8): 463–9.

Williams AE, Nester CJ, Ravey MI (2007) Rheumatoid arthritis patients' experiences of wearing therapeutic footwear - a qualitative investigation. *BMC Musculoskelet Disord.* 2007 Nov **1**; 8: 104.

Chapter 8

Comorbidity and complications of RA

Nicola Goodson and Raashid Luqmani

Key points

- Patients with rheumatoid arthritis have a reduced life expectancy
- The most common attributed cause of death in patients with RA is cardiovascular disease
- Infection, pulmonary, gastrointestinal and renal disease account for excess deaths in patients with RA compared to the general population
- Suppressing disease activity and reducing traditional cardiovascular risk factors may improve survival in RA
- Increased rates of infection, osteoporosis, depression respiratory, gastrointestinal and renal disease all contribute to the co-morbid disease burden in these patients
- Serious complications and co-morbid disease may cause rheumatological emergencies including: acute infection, cardiovascular events, peptic ulceration and gastrointestinal bleeding, cervical spine disease with spinal cord compression, lymphoproliferative malignancy, rheumatoid vasculitis and respiratory failure.

8.1 Introduction

Rheumatoid arthritis is associated with involvement of organ systems other than the joints and it is sometimes impossible to determine whether extra-articular disease complications in RA are due to the inflammatory process or due to associated comorbidity. Comorbidity may develop as a consequence of treatment of rheumatoid arthritis or indirectly as a consequence of developing arthritis. Associated comorbidity can serve as a major determinant of disease outcome in rheumatoid arthritis because of the effects on disability and increased risk of premature mortality.

The most frequently described complications in established rheumatoid arthritis include cardiovascular disease (CVD), respiratory disease, infection, osteoporosis, peptic ulcer disease, depression and lymphoproliferative malignancy.

8.2 Mortality in RA

Despite improvements in treatment, patients with RA still have a reduced life expectancy when compared to the general population. This equates to an average loss of 4–8 years of life. It is known that patients with RA have increased mortality, compared to the general population, from infections, renal disease, gastrointestinal disorders and lymphoproliferative disease. However these are responsible for only a small proportion of all deaths in patients with RA. Cardiovascular disease (CVD) is the most frequently identified cause of death (responsible for 35–50% of all deaths) as in the general population, but in RA it occurs about a decade earlier than in the general population.

8.3 Cardiovascular comorbidity

Structural cardiac lesions including pericarditis and non-specific mitral and aortic valve abnormalities are described in autopsy series and echocardiographic studies of RA patients. However, these lesions usually remain clinically silent and rarely lead to significant haemodynamic disturbances. These structural CVD features associated with RA do not appear to account for excess CVD mortality.

Increased CVD mortality rates have been observed in community-based cohorts of RA patients and in those with early inflammatory polyarthritis. This suggests that mechanisms which promote CVD mortality are not restricted to patients with severe RA but are also present early in the disease process.

Most studies have reported a 1.5–2 fold increase in events compared to the general population. Patients with RA are more likely to experience silent ischaemia and thus there is often a delay in seeking medical intervention. In addition, studies have demonstrated that RA patients are less likely to receive secondary CVD prevention with antiplatelet agents after a CVD event. These factors may contribute to the premature CVD mortality observed in RA patients.

Box 8.1 Avoiding cardiovascular morbidity in RA

- The co-prescription of ibuprofen and aspirin should be avoided because ibuprofen may reduce the antiplatelet effect of aspirin.
- Gastroprotection should be provided if aspirin is co-prescribed with non selective NSAIDs.
- ACE inhibitors should be used in patients who have heart failure.
- Patients with atherosclerotic cerebrovascular accidents should be managed with ACE inhibitors and thiazide diuretics in order to achieve tight blood pressure control with a target of <130/80 (see Table 8.1).
- Systemic inflammation may promote atherosclerotic CVD in RA. It is important to treat the arthritis effectively in order to minimize disease activity and reduce the inflammatory burden.

8.4 Risk factors for cardiovascular disease in RA

Possible explanations for the link between rheumatoid arthritis and premature atherosclerotic cardiovascular disease include shared risk factors for both conditions, e.g., cigarette smoking and obesity. Cigarette smoking increases both the risk of cardiovascular disease and the severity of arthritis. However, the cardiovascular risk in patients with rheumatoid arthritis cannot be entirely explained by an increased rate of traditional risk factors, suggesting that the disease itself or its treatment may be implicated. Chronic inflammation itself may promote atherosclerosis. There is increasing evidence that atherosclerosis is an inflammatory process. Patients with elevated inflammatory markers have a higher rate of cardiovascular events compared with patients who have lower inflammatory markers. Cardiovascular risk factors are modified by inflammatory disease activity. Box 8.1 outlines strategies to reduce cardiovascular events.

Therapies used to treat arthritis can influence cardiovascular risk, for good or ill. Use of DMARDs to achieve suppression of inflammatory disease appears to reduce the risk of CVD events in rheumatoid arthritis. Glucocorticoids may worsen the CVD risk profile by exacerbating hypertension, worsening dyslipidaemia and impairing glucose tolerance. By contrast, glucocorticoid use has been associated with paradoxical improvements in dyslipidaemia in rheumatoid arthritis. TNF-alpha antagonists are capable of modulating endothelial function and improving lipid profiles but may exacerbate existing congestive heart failure. Current recommendations suggest avoiding selective COX-2 inhibitors in patients with high cardiovascular risk. Lipid-lowering drugs (particularly statins) have been shown to have a moderate

Table 8.1 Medical interventions to reduce CVD in patients with RA

Medical interventions	Primary prevention of CVD if 10 year CVD risk is <20%	Primary prevention of CVD If 10 year CVD risk is ≥20%	Secondary prevention of CVD (known CVD, or known diabetes)
Lipid lowering therapy	Initiate treatment if:\n\nTotal cholesterol: HDL cholesterol ratio ≥6	Initiate lipid lowering therapy\n\nTarget values:\nTotal Cholesterol <5 mmol/L\nLDL cholesterol <3 mmol/L	Initiate lipid lowering therapy\n\nTarget values:\nTotal Cholesterol <4 mmol/L\nLDL cholesterol <2 mmol/L
Antihypertensives	Treat if hypertensive:\n\nTarget BP <140/90 mmHg	Treat if hypertensive:\n\nTarget BP <140/90 mmHg	Optimise BP\nTarget BP <130/80mmHg
Antiplatelet therapy*		Use antiplatelet agent if aged ≥ 50 years*	Use antiplatelet agent*

* Control elevated blood pressure first; Lifestyle interventions to promote health are recommended for all patients as well as treatment for diabetes mellitus if present.

effect in reducing inflammation among patients with rheumatoid arthritis and may achieve additional reduction in CVD events by this pleiotropic effect. Table 8.1 summarizes preventive measures to reduce cardiovascular morbidity in patients with RA.

8.5 Osteoporosis and rheumatoid arthritis

Osteoporosis and bone fracture are a major cause of morbidity in patients with rheumatoid arthritis. Juxta-articular osteopenia (Figure 8.1) and generalized bone loss occur early in RA and there is a 2 fold increased risk of both hip fracture and symptomatic vertebral fractures in patients with established RA compared to the general population. Osteoporotic fractures are associated with disability, mortality and major financial and social impact as well as leading to significant decline in quality of life. The causes of osteoporosis associated with rheumatoid arthritis are multifactorial and are shown in Table 8.2.

8.6 Prevention of osteoporosis

Lifestyle factors such as regular weight-bearing exercise and adequate dietary calcium and vitamin D intake are recommended for all patients to help to prevent deterioration of bone mineral density (BMD).

Figure 8.1 X-ray of Juxtarticular osteopenia in RA

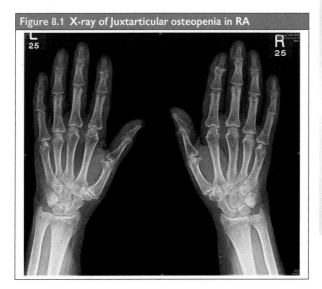

Table 8.2 Causes of adverse bone health in RA

Causes of adverse bone health in RA	Mechanisms
Chronic inflammation	Proinflammatory cytokines • Activate osteoclasts • Mediate bone loss
Treatment effects	High dose prolonged use of glucocorticoids • Inhibit calcium resorption • Increase renal calcium excretion • Inhibit new bone formation.
Lifestyle	Lack of exercise • Reduced mobility • Reduce weight bearing activity • Promotes bone loss

Note: Reduction of systemic inflammation by the use of low dose glucocorticoids may have a beneficial effect on bone mineral density. However, high dose prolonged use of glucocorticoid results in bone loss. In addition, reduction in physical ability and reduced weight-bearing activity will also contribute to loss of bone in RA.

Primary fracture prevention, using bisphosphonates (or strontium ranelate, if intolerant to bisphosphonates), is recommended for post menopausal females who have reduced bone mineral density (BMD) (T score <–2.5), measured using Dual Energy X-ray Absorbtiometry (DEXA) (Figure 8.2). If patients are older than age 70 and have had a fracture or at least 3 independent risk factors for osteoporosis, they should be treated without the need for DEXA imaging. Independent risk factors for osteoporotic fracture include parental history of hip fracture, alcohol intake of more than 4 units/day and established rheumatoid arthritis. Other indicators of low BMD include low body mass index (defined as less than 22 kg/m^2) and medical conditions such as ankylosing spondylitis, Crohn's disease, conditions that cause prolonged immobility, untreated premature menopause.

The use of glucocorticoids is associated with an increased risk of fragility fracture over and above the effect of lowering bone mineral density. Because loss of BMD is greatest in the first few months of

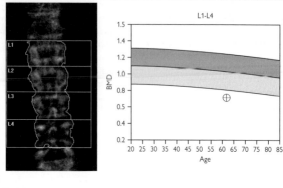

Figure 8.2 **DEXA** scan showing typical results in a patient with RA who also has osteoporosis: note that the patients's total T score is less than 2.5 standard deviations below the average

Results Summary:

Region	Area[cm2]	BMC[(g)]	BMD[(g/cm2)]	T-score	PR (Peak Reference)	Z-score	AM (Age Matched)
L1	17.25	13.34	0.773	–2.7	72	–2.1	77
L2	17.89	12.60	0.746	–3.2	68	–2.5	73
L3	17.72	12.64	0.713	–3.5	65	–2.9	69
L4	18.84	11.87	0.630	–4.2	58	–3.5	62
Total	70.70	50.45	0.714	–3.4	65	–2.8	70

glucocorticoid therapy, it is important to consider early use of bone protective medication in patients who begin taking oral steroids with anticipated use for longer than 3 months. Royal College of Physicians (London) guidelines recommend that, in addition to general measures to limit bone loss, specific medication to prevent glucocorticoid induced osteoporosis should be initiated in all patients aged 65 years or older on prolonged steroid treatment. In younger patients, DEXA measurement of bone mineral density should be used to guide treatment. Patients with T-scores of −1.5 or less should receive specific treatment.

8.7 Depression and rheumatoid arthritis

Patients with RA are twice as likely to suffer from depression as members of the general population. Hospital based studies report severe depression in up to 40% of patients with rheumatoid arthritis. Depression complicating RA is associated with increased levels of disability. There is an association between the severity of depression and functional disability, particularly during the early years of RA. Depression contributes to both the level of disability and work disability in patients with inflammatory joint disease. Depression in RA is associated with higher levels of fatigue and sleep disturbance and depressed patients with RA have higher levels of T-cell activation which may predispose them to more severe disease manifestations. These patients are also likely to have a reduced life expectancy. Patients with rheumatoid arthritis and depression are more likely to develop cardiovascular disease.

Treatment of depression in established RA is based on standard therapies. However, there is evidence that in the patient with RA, depression is less responsive to antidepressant therapy or combined antidepressant plus cognitive behavioural therapy compared with depressed patients who do not have arthritis.

8.8 Gastrointestinal tract disease and rheumatoid arthritis

Peptic ulcer disease is more common in RA. This reflects the effect of treatment rather than the disease process. Non-steroidal anti-inflammatory drugs (NSAIDs) increase the risk of peptic ulceration; this effect is strongly potentiated when glucocorticoids are also given. Peptic ulceration can be asymptomatic in RA. In addition small bowel ulceration has been described in association with long term NSAID use. Current guidelines recommend that long term use of NSAIDs should be avoided where possible and that gastroprotection should be provided for those patients who require long-term NSAIDs.

Table 8.3 Prevention and treatment of osteoporosis

General measures to reduce risk of osteoporosis	Medication licensed for prevention of osteoporosis and fracture
• Reduce dose of oral glucocorticoid and consider glucocorticoid-sparing therapy • Optimize calcium and vitamin D intake, either by dietary modification or by use of calcium and vitamin D containing supplements • Regular weight bearing exercise • Avoid tobacco use and alcohol abuse • Optimize body weight • Assess falls risk	Calcium/vitamin D (1000–1200mg/800 IU) • All patients on oral steriods • May increase muscle strength, decrease body sway, decrease falls Bisphosphonates Strontium ranelate Raloxifene Teriparatide • Daily subcutaneous injection for 18 months • Secondary care use in women ≥65 years only at present Hormone replacement therapy (HRT) (Women) • Reduces fracture risk at all sites • Increases risk of breast cancer, coronary heart disease (CHD), stroke and dementia • Not recommended for long-term use

8.9 Infection and rheumatoid arthritis

Infection is a major cause of morbidity and mortality in rheumatoid arthritis. Patients are particularly prone to pulmonary infection, generalized sepsis, osteomyelitis, cellulitis and septic arthritis (see Box 8.2). Rates of hospitalisation for infection are increased in patients with rheumatoid arthritis compared to the general population. RA and its treatment are both associated with increased infection risk. Patients with RA have disturbed cellular immunity with impaired T-suppressor and natural killer cell function which may predispose them to infection. In addition, the use of glucocorticoids, DMARDs and biologic therapies have the potential to increase infection risk through their immune modulating effects. However, it is important to note that the doses of methotrexate used to treat RA are anti-inflammatory rather than immunosuppressive.

8.10 Respiratory infection

Rates of respiratory infection are increased in patients with RA. Indeed, serious infection rates in RA (defined as infection leading to hospital admission, use of intravenous antibiotics or death) are

> **Box 8.2 Management of patients with suspected septic arthritis**
>
> - Joint aspiration and microbiological examination of joint fluid is mandatory for making a diagnosis
> - Patients should usually be admitted to hospital
> - Antibiotics should not be started prior to joint aspiration
> - A possibly infected prosthetic joint should always be referred to an orthopaedic surgeon for aspiration in a sterile setting.
> - Blood tests should include cultures, FBC CRP ESR and renal function
> - Biologic therapies should be stopped and temporary withdrawal of DMARDs may be required.
> - Parenteral or intra-articular glucocorticoids should be avoided
> - Long-term oral glucocorticoids should be continued to prevent acute adrenal insufficiency.
> - Use of repeated aspiration or arthroscopic washout of the infected joint may be required.
> - Treatment is usually prolonged requiring at least 2 weeks of intravenous antibiotics followed by a further 4 weeks of oral antibiotics.

2–3 times that of the general population. Several factors associated with RA contribute to the increased risk of serious respiratory infection. These include the effect of RA on the immune system, the use of immunosuppressive medication and corticosteroids, increased rates of cigarette smoking and the frailty and disability associated with established disease. The recognition that patients are at high risk of respiratory infection has lead to the recommendation that they should receive vaccination against pneumococcal capsular antigens and annual influenza vaccination.

8.11 **Infection and RA medication**

Immunosuppressive therapy may exacerbate and mask infection, and temporary withdrawal is strongly advised during active infection. Any agent that suppresses the immune system may increase the severity of any concurrent infection. Glucocorticoids should not be stopped if the patient has been taking them for a prolonged period, because of concerns over adrenal insufficiency; however, we recommend that all patients should have a cautious reduction of glucocorticoids to the lowest level required, if necessary supplemented by a higher dose of DMARD treatment. It is unusual that a patient requires treatment with more than 5 mg/day of prednisolone over extended periods.

Biologic agents which suppress inflammation inherently render the host more susceptible to infection. There is an increased rate of bacterial intracellular infections including tuberculosis (TB) in patients receiving anti-TNFα therapy. It is important to test for and treat latent TB infections prior to starting biologic treatments for RA. In addition, anti-TNFα agents are associated with higher rates of serious skin and soft tissue infections than conventional DMARDs.

Prior to any planned surgery, it is important to discuss withdrawal of immunosuppressive medications. In most cases, there is no compelling evidence to stop therapy. For high infection risk procedures, such as joint replacement, anti-TNFα drugs are usually withdrawn 2–4 weeks prior to surgery. Patients should be closely monitored for infection because anti-TNFα treatment may mask typical signs. Anti TNFα therapy can be restarted 3 weeks post surgery when incisions have healed. Other DMARDs can usually be continued throughout the perioperative period if there are no concerns over sepsis or wound healing.

8.12 Joint sepsis

Rheumatoid arthritis is a risk factor for septic arthritis. This risk is highest in patients with severe longstanding seropositive RA and is more common in patients treated with glucocorticoids. The clinical presentation is often atypical. In 25% of cases, the infection is polyarticular and associated with a poor prognosis including a mortality rate of nearly 50%. Staphylococcus aureus is responsible for more than two-thirds of identified infections, with streptococci and gram-negative bacilli next in frequency. Streptococcus pneumoniae causes 5% of all cases of septic arthritis and is associated with polyarticular infections. The most common site is the knee, followed by the hip and shoulder.

8.13 Prosthetic joint infection

Rheumatoid arthritis is a risk factor for infection in prosthetic joints. Patients with RA have a 1.8 fold increased risk of requiring arthroplasty revision because of infection, compared to OA patients. It is important to distinguish between chronic infection due to intraoperative contamination, resulting in septic loosening, and acute haematogenous infection, because in the latter, emergency treatment can salvage the prosthesis. Identification of the organism in the joint is the key to the diagnosis. Joint aspiration should be performed as an emergency by an orthopaedic surgeon in an aseptic environment. Antibiotics should be initiated after microbiological specimens have been collected. In the case of early infection or acute haematogenous infection, a thorough debridement with synovectomy may save a well-fixed prosthesis. In chronic infections, it is often necessary to remove the prosthesis, the cement and all devitalized tissue in order to heal the infection, due to the formation of a biofilm.

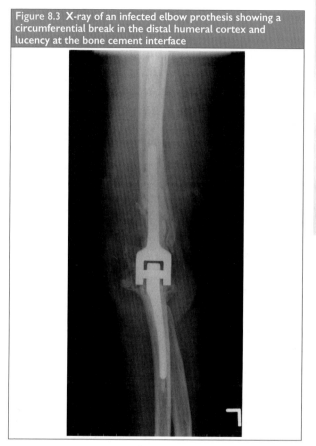

Figure 8.3 **X-ray of an infected elbow prothesis showing a circumferential break in the distal humeral cortex and lucency at the bone cement interface**

8.14 **Immunizations/vaccinations**

8.14.1 **Live vaccines**

Live vaccines use an attenuated live pathogen to achieve active immunization. Commonly used live vaccines include measles, mumps and rubella (MMR), BCG, varicella vaccination, yellow fever and Japanese encephalitis vaccinations. The Sabin oral live polio vaccine is no longer routinely used.

Patients receiving medication are recommended to avoid receiving live vaccines, but it is not entirely clear whether or not low-dose weekly methotrexate (as used for RA) and/or low-dose daily glucocorticoid preclude the use of live vaccines. It is recommended that these medications should be stopped at least 3 months (longer with leflunomide because of long half life) before live vaccines are administered. A period of 3–4 weeks is required after live vaccination prior to starting immunosuppressant or cytotoxic drugs. If a significant high risk contact occurs in an immunosuppressed patient not known to have prior immunity, specific pooled human immunoglobulins should be considered, for example zoster immune globulin after exposure to varicella zoster, or immunoglobulins (IVIg) after exposure to measles.

8.14.2 Inactivated toxoid or subcomponent vaccines

Vaccines that are prepared either from inactivated virus, bacteria, or extracts of detoxified exotoxins can be used in patients receiving cytotoxic or immunosuppressive therapy. However, in immunosuppressed patients the immunological response to inactivated vaccines may not be as strong as that in the general population. More frequent boosters may be required to generate an adequate immune response.

8.14.3 Rituximab

Patients treated with rituximab should not receive active immunization during B-cell depletion. Live vaccines should not be used, and inactivated toxoid or subcomponent vaccines are likely to be less effective because antibody-producing B-cells will be depleted and patients are less likely to mount an adequate immune response. Ideally, immunization with inactivated vaccines should occur 2–4 weeks prior to initiating rituximab or in-between courses when the B-cell counts have returned to the normal range.

Table 8.5 Commonly used vaccines

Live attenuated vaccines	Inactivated vaccines
Measles	Diphtheria
Mumps	Haemophilus influenzae type b
Rubella	Hepatitis A
Varicella zoster	Hepatitis B
BCG	Influenza
Polio (oral)	Meningococcal
Typhoid (oral)	Pertussis
Yellow fever	Pneumococcal
	Poliomyelitis
	Tetanus
	Typhoid

8.15 Extra-articular disease in RA

RA is a systemic disease, with its predominant manifestations in the joints. Careful inspection of the hands may reveal a few trivial nail edge infarcts (Figure 8.4), representing a minor manifestation of rheumatoid vasculitis. However, many patients experience systemic effects when the disease is active (see Table 8.6). These include fatigue and weight loss, and in severe cases fever, lymphadenopathy, splenomegaly, and hepatomegaly. Most of these manifestations resolve with control of systemic inflammation through the use of standard treatment for the arthritis, such as methotrexate.

Rheumatoid nodules (Figure 8.5) occur in up to 20% of patients, although previously they were more commonly seen. They are chronic granulomata and are usually of no clinical consequence. Although they typically appear following the onset of the disease, they may occur

Table 8.6 Extra-articular features of RA

Systemic	Weight loss, fever, tiredness, lymphadenopathy
Haematological	Anaemia of chronic disease; thrombocytopenia and neutropenia with splenomegaly (Felty's syndrome)
Cutaneous	Nail edge infarcts/splinter haemorrhages, leg ulcers, nodules
Mucous membranes/eyes	Dry eyes and dry mouth
Ear, nose and throat	Hearing loss (rare) due to vasculitis; cricoarytenoid involvement (rare) due to active arthritis
Respiratory	Interstitial pneumonitis, pulmonary fibrosis, bronchiolitis obliterans, pleural effusion and bronchiectasis
Cardiovascular	Pericarditis (acute or chronic), myocarditis, conduction defects, valvular heart disease; aortitis
Gastrointestinal	Amyloid of the gut resulting in malabsorption and or diarrhoea
Renal	Proteinuria, and rarely renal failure due to amyloidosis; vasculitis of the kidney
Neurological	Entrapment neuropathy e.g. carpal tunnel syndrome; peripheral sensory neuropathy, mononeuritis multiplex, cervical cord compression due to unstable cervical spine
Malignancy	Increased risk of tumours especially B cell lymphoma (this risk is slightly worsened by the use of immunosuppressive agents)
Other immunological diseases	Increased incidence of thyroid disease

Figure 8.4 Fingers in a patient with RA who has asymptomatic nail edge infarcts

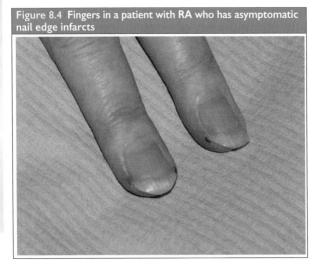

Figure 8.5 Rheumatoid nodules in a large olecranon bursa overlying the elbow of a patient with RA

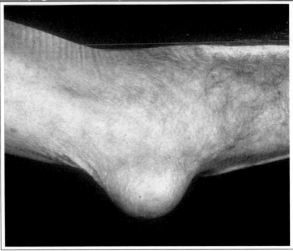

prior to the development of arthritis (and if they occur in the lung, they may be mistaken for a lung tumour). Some drugs such as methotrexate may actually accelerate nodule formation even while improving the arthritis. Surgical removal of nodules is straightforward, but there is a high risk of recurrence.

In longstanding, untreated systemic inflammation of any type, there is a risk of developing secondary amyloidosis due to the excess formation of amyloid proteins, which are deposited in organs such as the kidney, heart and gut, interfering with normal function. Amyloidosis was particularly common in Finland, but the incidence is falling, possibly as a result of better treatment of the underlying inflammatory disease. However, amyloidosis should be suspected in patients with longstanding RA who develop organ impairment, which cannot be attributed to their current drug therapy.

Patients with RA commonly complain of dry, gritty eyes, or dry mouth. The presence of sicca syndrome is common and reflects the systemic inflammatory effects of the disease, resulting in inflammation of salivary and lachrymal glands reducing their exocrine function.

8.16 Pulmonary manifestations of rheumatoid arthritis

Lung involvement in RA is common, but not always serious (see Table 8.7). If patients are examined by high resolution CT scanning of the lung, most will have some abnormalities, especially those with long standing disease (Figure 8.6). However, for many patients this does not have serious clinical consequences.

Pleural involvement with effusion and pleural inflammation is the most common pulmonary manifestation of RA, found in 40–70% of patients at autopsy. It is symptomatic in only about 10% of RA patients and is more common in males with severe seropositive disease. Whilst bronchiectasis is a frequent finding on High Resolution Computerised Tomography (HRCT) scanning of rheumatoid lungs (Figure 8.7), it remains asymptomatic in the majority of patients. Bronchiolar disease with bronchiolitis obliterans can be a cause of chronic cough and dyspnoea in RA. This is usually associated with an obstructive pattern on pulmonary function testing.

Table 8.7 Pulmonary manifestations of rheumatoid arthritis

Lung structure	Pathology
Pleura	Pleural effusion/pleuritis
Airway	Cricoarytenoid arthritis Bronchiectasis Bronchiolitis obliterans (also involves the lung parenchyma)
Parenchyma	Interstitial pneumonitis (NSIP or UIP) pulmonary fibrosis (honeycomb lung), rheumatoid lung nodules, infection
Respiratory muscles	Drug induced pneumonitis Diaphragmatic and respiratory mucle weakness
Pulmonary vasculature	Pulmonary hypertension

Figure 8.6 **HRCT scanning of the lung shows asymptomatic ground-glass opacities in the lung parenchyma (present in more than 90% of patients with longstanding RA)**

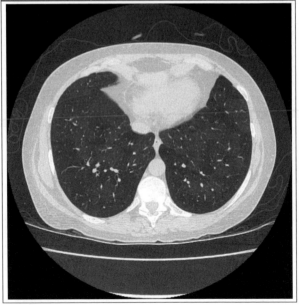

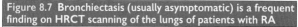

Figure 8.7 Bronchiectasis (usually asymptomatic) is a frequent finding on HRCT scanning of the lungs of patients with RA

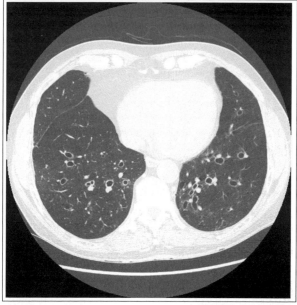

Idiopathic lung inflammation (interstitial pneumonitis) in RA, unrelated to any drug reaction, is occasionally progressive. Interstitial pneumonitis can be classified into several types, based on histology of the pulmonary lesion. In RA the 2 main types are non specific intertitial pneumonia (NSIP) (Figure 8.8), and usual intertitial pneumonia (UIP) (Figure 8.9). There is controversy over the use of methotrexate and azathioprine treatment in patients with UIP or NSIP, due to concern that the drugs may make the lung disease worse, but there is no good evidence to support this. NSIP is often steroid responsive, whereas UIP is more resistant. Use of chemotherapy such as cyclophosphamide may be considered in such cases, under specialist advice. Interstitial lung disease leading to pulmonary fibrosis carries a poor prognosis in RA. Studies conducted 20 years ago demonstrated a median of survival of only 4 years after diagnosis of pulmonary fibrosis in RA. Plain chest radiographs are usually normal and HRCT scanning is required to investigate this. However HRCT would be recommended only if patients are experiencing symptoms, and have evidence of abnormal gas transfer on lung function testing.

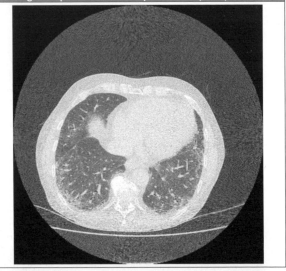

Figure 8.8 HRCT scan of lungs from a patient with RA showing non specific interstitial pneumonia (NSIP)

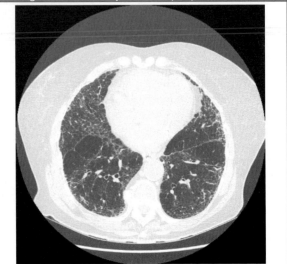

Figure 8.9 HRCT scan of lungs from a patient with RA showing usual interstitial pneumonia (UIP)

The most common finding is usual interstitial pneumonia (UIP). These patients do not usually respond to high doses of corticosteroids, and have a worse prognosis. Single or multiple rheumatoid nodules may occur in the lung parenchyma (Figure 8.10).

Lung disease has been associated with several drugs used to treat RA. In particular methotrexate pneumonitis is identified as a rheumatological emergency. Fortunately this is a rare side effect of this drug only occurring in <1% of those treated, particularly with concurrent folic acid. Symptoms of methotrexate pneumonitis are very similar to that of an acute respiratory infection, with a dry cough, breathlessness and pyrexia, and diagnosis is often difficult. Other drugs that have been associated with interstitial pneumonitis include leflunomide, intramuscular gold and with the use of anti-TNFα therapy in a few case reports.

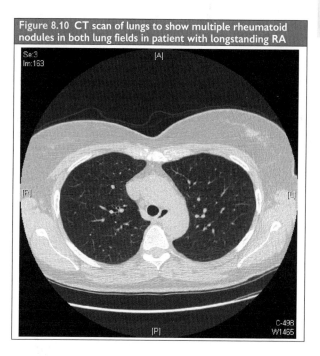

Figure 8.10 CT scan of lungs to show multiple rheumatoid nodules in both lung fields in patient with longstanding RA

8.17 **Renal disease and rheumatoid arthritis**

Apart from amyloid, the kidney can be involved directly by the rheumatoid disease, but this is unusual. More likely the drugs used to manage RA can be nephrotoxic. Typically the use of NSAIDs may be associated with the development of hypertension and in some cases with tubular interstitial nephritis. In very rare cases, a necrotizing vasculitis of the kidney may present with sudden deterioration in renal function and typically associated with microscopic haematuria and proteinuria. Analgesic nephropathy is rare but still occasionally seen in patients using excess amounts of paracetamol for joint pain.

8.18 **Vasculitis and rheumatoid arthritis**

The spectrum of inflammation may include vasculitis, which rarely gives rise to significant clinical manifestations. Lip gland biopsy studies and post mortem examinations show sub clinical vasculitis to be present in a third of patients. The most common clinical feature is the finding of small skin infarcts, manifest as nail edge lesions, splinter haemorrhages or "flea bite" lesions on the hands or feet, or over the surface of nodules. The majority of these patients do not require any specific therapy, other than control of their joint disease.

A small number of patients may have features of multi system vasculitis as part of their RA; typically this occurs in patients with established disease for more than 10 years; manifestations include those of a systemic vasculitis – mononeuritis multiplex, gut infarction, leg ulceration (Figure 8.11) and proliferative glomerulonephritis. All sizes of vessel can be involved, and any vascular bed can be affected. Cytotoxic drugs and steroids are indicated for more severe manifestations as shown in Table 8.8.

8.19 **Neurological complications of rheumatoid arthritis**

Entrapment neuropathies may occur in RA as a result of nerve compression by expanding synovial tissue. At the wrist, median nerve compression results in transient or persistent carpal tunnel symptoms. These features may resolve with treatment of the underlying synovitis. Otherwise, they may require direct treatment, either with a local glucocorticoid injection, or surgical decompression.

Rheumatoid arthritis frequently affects the cervical spine of patients with very longstanding disease. Whilst most cervical spine disease can be managed conservatively, instability of the neck can lead to progressive myelopathy and neurological damage. Atlantoaxial subluxation is

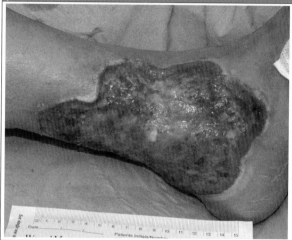

Figure 8.11 Skin vasculitis resulting in leg ulceration in a patient with RA

Table 8.8 Treatment of vasculitis in rheumatoid disease

Severity	Clinical features	Therapy
Mild	Nail edge infarcts, flea bite lesions, splinter haemorrhages	No specific treatment required
Moderate	Deep cutaneous ulcers , in the absence of arterial or venous insufficiency	Steroids and cyclophosphamide, plus iv prostacyclin; may require skin grafting in severe cases infection risk is high
Severe	Critical organ or multi-organ involvement e.g. mononeuritis multiplex, gut infarction	Steroids and cyclophosphamide. Infection risk is high

the most common form of cervical spine instability seen in rheumatoid arthritis. This commonly gives rise to local pain and stiffness but may progress asymptomatically in some patients.

The risk of progressive myelopathy increases once the distance between the anterior body of C2 and the anterior arch of the C1 vertebra is greater than 9 mm. The development of new neurological symptoms and signs in a patient with RA represents a rheumatological emergency that requires prompt investigation and treatment.

Neurosurgical decompression can prevent further neurological deterioration but the risk of operating on a potentially osteoporotic cervical spine in an immunosuppressed patients with associated comorbidity makes surgery a high risk procedure (see Chapter 9).

Further reading

Chakravarty K *et al.* (2008) BSR/BHPR guideline for disease-modifying anti-rheumatic drug (DMARD) therapy in consultation with the British Association of Dermatologists. *Rheumatology* (Oxford): in Press

Luqmani RA, *et al.* (2009) British Society for Rheumatology & British Health Professionals in Rheumatology Guideline for the management of rheumatoid arthritis (after the first 2 years). *Rheumatology* (Oxford): doi 10.1093/rheumatology/ken450a.

Naninni C, *et al* (2008). Lung disease in rheumatoid arthritis. *Curr Opin Rheumatol* (3) 340–6.

Royal College of Physicians, Bone and Tooth Society of Great Britain (2001). Osteoporosis—Clinical guidelines for prevention and treatment—Update on pharmacological interventions and an algorithm for management. Working Party Report. London: Royal College of Physicians.

Chapter 9

Surgical management of rheumatoid arthritis: introduction and spinal involvement

Tom Cadoux-Hudson, Hemant Pandit, Ian McNab, Raashid Luqmani

Key points

- Reconstructive surgery should be undertaken before the patient becomes severely incapacitated
- Patients should be as fit as possible, with optimal synovitis control, correction of blood dyscrasia and adequate nutrition (normal albumin)
- Active disease is not a contraindication to surgery, nor is use of corticosteroids and methotrexate
- Mild atlanto-axial subluxation is present in 30% at diagnosis of RA. Progression is usually associated with neck pain, brachalgia and myelopathy
- Progressive myelopathy is most likely to occur if the PADI (Posterior atlanto-dens interval) is 13 mm or less.
- Soft collars are of little biomechanical use. They remind the patient that they have a neck problem, which may indirectly limit spinal cord damage
- Delayed diagnosis of myelopathy, often associated with deformity such as basilar invagination or kyphosis, requires more complex and hazardous surgery.

9.1 Introduction

The main treatment of inflammatory joint disease is medical control of synovitis. However, once irreversible joint damage has occurred, reconstructive surgical treatment is indicated and should be undertaken

Box 9.1 **Investigations prior to surgery**

- Plain X-ray (usually suffices)
- MRI
- MRI arthrogram (especially in the hip joint)
- Biopsy

before the patient becomes severely incapacitated. Box 9.1 lists investigations that may be required prior to surgery.

9.2 **Operative treatment**

The patient should be as fit as possible, ideally with synovitis under good medical control and no chest, urinary or skin infection. Care must be taken perioperatively with renal function, hydration and steroid requirements.

Surgical treatment forms only a part of the continuing management of the patient by the whole medical team. Active disease is not a contraindication to surgery, nor is the use of methotrexate or glucocorticoid; a temporary increase in the dosage of the latter may be required in the perioperative period.

The ultimate successful outcome of surgery for patients is determined not just by matching the correct patient to the correct procedure and meticulous attention to surgical detail and technique, but also by the dedicated work of the nurses, physiotherapists, occupational therapists, and patients themselves, during their postoperative rehabilitation (See Box 9.2).

The order of procedures should be tailored to the individual. The operations most likely to be successful are usually performed first, in order to build confidence with the patient. It is probably advantageous to correct the lower limb abnormalities before addressing upper limb problems. On the other hand, problems in the upper limb may impair rehabilitation following lower limb surgery (it is difficult to use a frame or crutches in the presence of severe arthritis in the hands and wrists and therefore becomes a priority). In patients who require intubation, clinical and radiographic assessment of cervical spine mobility and stability is essential. Patients are susceptible to perioperative compression neuropathies of superficial nerves. Perioperative management of drug therapy should be individually tailored on a careful balance of risks and benefits.

A recommended order of reconstruction would be the forefoot, hip, knee, followed by the hind foot and ankle. However, it is important to consider the patient's most debilitating and/or deformed joints.

> **Box 9.2 Peri-operative issues associated with RA**
>
> - Timing of surgery in relation to medical treatment and control of arthritis (preferably optimal with DMARDs which should usually be continued)
> - Use of immunosuppressant and/or steroids increasing the risk of infection
> - Past medical history, general health, treatment history
> - Cardiovascular and respiratory assessment, poor jaw mobility, micrognathia, reduced lung capacity, cervical spine movements including imaging to exclude subluxation to anticipate anaesthetic problems
> - Walking ability and use of suitable walking aids, presence of significant lower limb problems, thoraco lumbar spine problems
> - Skin conditions (including ulcers or thin skin)
> - Presence of and treatment of vasculitis
> - Presence of and treatment of osteoporosis
> - Chronic anaemia
> - Polyarticular involvement with contractures – positioning and padding to prevent pressure sores
> - Home environment, and functional abilities and requirements
> - Optimise occupational therapy, physiotherapy, splints and aids.

9.3 Cervical spine problems in RA

Rheumatoid arthritis of the cervical spine has been a great challenge both in terms of diagnosis and treatment. The axial joints (occipito-cervical; C0/C1 and atlanto-axial; C1/C2) and sub-axial facet joints all contain synovial tissue; the time and pattern of presentation varies. 30% of patients will have radiological evidence of subluxation at C1/C2 at diagnosis. The majority of these patients will not progress and will not require surgery. The challenge is to select and manage those patients who have either developed or are likely to develop brachiomyelopathy. Clinical cervical spine involvement is seen in patients with longstanding disease, typically greater than 8 years. The presence of neck pain is a common feature. Classic symptoms and signs of established cervical myelopathy can be confused in the presence of stiff, painful joints, peripheral neuropathies and myopathies.

Medical therapy remains the mainstay of disease management. Conservative management of the cervical spine includes the effective use of DMARDs to control synovitis, analgesia, local nerve blocks, heat treatment, TENs machines, relaxation techniques for symptom relief. Pain may extend from the neck down into the shoulders and up to the skull because of muscle spasm and weakness. Exercise can increase muscle strength and reduce some of these symptoms.

The reduced use of corticosteroids and early use of immunosuppressive drugs has dramatically improved bone quality. The erosive nature of synovitis is better contained and surgical outcomes improved, because a more focussed surgical approach is possible.

The cervical spinal cord does not tolerate compression or contusion. Surgery is aimed at halting further neurological deterioration. Axial disorders present with neck pain (C2 nerve root irritation/compression) and can be extremely disabling, occasionally leading to suicide. Sub-axial disorders in RA behave in a more aggressive but similar way to more common degenerative disorders of disc and facet joint pathology. Surgery involves anterior cervical discectomy for disc prolapse supported by cage implant and anterior plating.

Osteoporosis and facet joint destruction can lead to deformities requiring extensive reconstruction.

9.3.1 **Axial disorders**

The occipital condyle to lateral mass C1 joint is usually robust and unlikely to be involved unless there is significant synovial destruction and flattening of the articular surface leading to subluxation and rotational deformities.

The atlanto-axial joint is commonly involved in RA due to laxity of the transverse ligament (as a result of pannus formation and intrinsic changes in the ligament) and bone erosion. Subluxation occurs when pannus invades the synovial joint anterior to the odontoid peg and posterior to the anterior arch of CI (Figure 9.1). Pannus exerts a profound effect on the otherwise immensely strong transverse ligament (breaking strain of 350N). Expansion between C1 and C2 leads to eventual failure, exposing the cord to contusional injury and eventually to frank compression (Figure 9.2). The clinical effect is seen as increased tone in the limbs (cervical myelopathy). Myelopathy is an adaptive process which can be masked by minor lower motor neurone pathologies commonly present in patients with long-standing disease, in which peripheral nerves attempt to pass damaged peripheral small joints. Severe cord damage can develop without traditional signs of myelopathy.

Plain dynamic (flexion and extension) X-rays can be used to assess movement at C1/ C2 but posterior atlanto-dens interval (PADI) is a more effective predictor of myelopathy in 70–80% of patients (Figure 9.3). This assumes that the average spinal cord diameter is 11–12mm and PADI of 13 mm or less would result in contusional injury followed by compression.

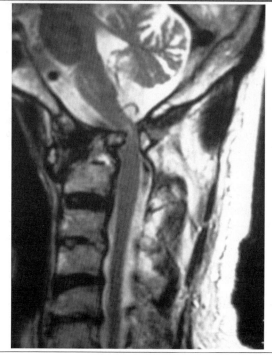

Figure 9.1 **MRI showing atlanto axial subluxation as pannus invades the synovial joint anterior to the odontoid peg and posterior to the anterior arch of CI**

The anterior atlanto-dens interval (AADI) is the distance between the posterior surface of anterior atlas and anterior surface of dens. Although a distance of more than 3 mm in adults is abnormal, it is less reliable than the PADI, because it does not take into account the pre-existing spinal cord diameter.

Abnormal movement which is threatening the cord can be controlled by fusion. Bone grafts and wiring achieved moderate success (60% control of disease process). Poor fusion rates were associated with poor bone quality and reliance on corticosteroids to control synovitis. More recent techniques have focused on achieving stronger initial fusion such as lateral mass C1/C2 screw fusion with less reliance on bone grafting (Figure 9.4). These have produced better results with shorter hospital stays and less need for post-operative external fixation.

Figure 9.2 Expansion between C1 and C2 has lead to frank compression of the cord in a patient with RA

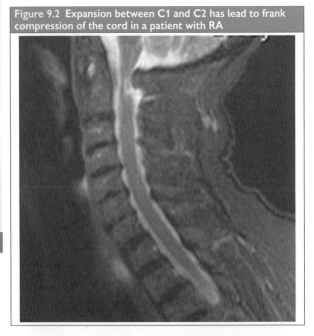

Figure 9.3 Lateral cervical spine X-ray to show posterior atlanto-dens interval (PADI)

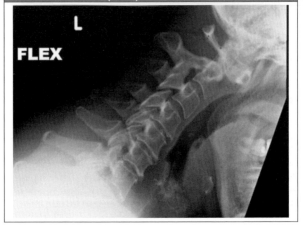

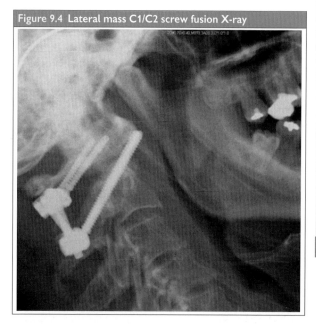

Figure 9.4 Lateral mass C1/C2 screw fusion X-ray

Basilar invagination occurs because subluxation and erosion allows the dens to migrate through the foramen magnum and threaten the brain stem (Figure 9.5). Advanced cases require transoral resection of the odontoid peg. The posterior fusion often has to be more widespread (Typical C0 to C5 or below), which is an extensive procedure for patients. The end result is long term restriction in neck movement and risk of further surgery to the lower cervicothoracic levels. Occasionally this process of erosion of the dens weakens the cortical surface leaving the dens vulnerable to fracture. This diagnosis can be easily missed on plain X-rays because the anterior arch of C1 moves with upper part of C2.

9.3.2 Sub-axial disorder

The formation of pannus, characteristic of the more mobile C1/C2 is less common in the subaxial spine. Bone destruction in the lateral mass and lamina can lead to disc pathology, reduction in disc height and impaction of the lower lamina into the upper level, causing gradual cord compression and myelopathy with loss of proprioception because the dorsal columns become more contused and compressed. The anterior displacement of the upper vertebra also contributes to the 'stair case' appearance of the sub-axial spine (Figure 9.6).

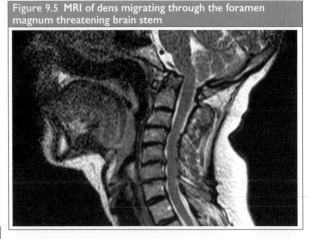

Figure 9.5 MRI of dens migrating through the foramen magnum threatening brain stem

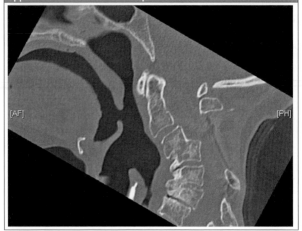

Figure 9.6 Lateral cervical spine X ray to show the 'stair case' appearance of the sub-axial spine

Loss of nucleus pulposus may be followed by rapid stabilisation and fusion at several levels. Osteophyte formation can improve load-bearing in the presence of ligamental laxity but can also cause brachalgia and neck pain. In most circumstances the osteophytes aid stability and lead to fusion. Nerve root compression can be mistaken for elbow joint pain (C7 nerve root) or thumb PIP disorder (C6). 80% of disc prolapses heal spontaneously with partial or complete fusion. The process usually starts at C5/6 or C6/7. However the upper levels (C3/4 and C4/5) may not fuse and the resultant cord compression may be difficult to diagnose. This ascending disc pathology with partial healing is characteristic of the cervical spine in RA, sometimes presenting in a 'step like' fashion with the appearance of a 'stair case' (see Figure 9.6). Conservative treatment is recommended where the symptoms are mild and imaging shows a generous spinal cord diameter (more than 14 mm). Surgical intervention is aimed at dealing with the symptomatic disc via an anterior cervical discectomy and fusion.

RA leads to progressive erosion of the synovial membrane and cartilage, leaving the cortical surface of the facet joints vulnerable to erosion and subluxation. Facet joint disorder in its mildest form is almost uniformly present. This process may occur at several levels leading to a 'stair case' neck. Neurological compression will occur early if the natural diameter of the spinal canal is narrow.

Bone quality is reduced due to active systemic disease and prolonged glucocorticoid administration leading to vertebral body collapse. The lateral masses and pedicles are usually preserved resulting in forward angulation (kyphosis). This may exacerbate any disc or facet joint disorder.

Erosive disease involves a combination of disc, facet, ligamental and bone mineral structural problems. The kyphotic and occasional scoliotic deformities can be a major surgical challenge. With modern anterior expandable cage implants and posterior lateral mass poly axial screw and rod implants these deformities can usually be treated with excellent results.

9.4 Incidence

In RA, there has been a reduction in the incidence of erosive disease, but the ligamentous laxity remains a problem and represents the major indication for surgical intervention at the axial level (C1/C2 subluxation). Minimally invasive surgical techniques have been developed. Sub-axial disease has also become less common with better medical care, and reduced use of glucocorticoid has helped to preserve cortical bone structure.

9.5 Pathophysiology

The major spinal ligaments (transverse and apical) are deranged early in a significant minority of patients. 30% have asymptomatic subluxation at C1/C2 or more than 3 mm on flexion/extension cervical spine

X-rays, which represents a risk to the spinal cord. However, there is only limited capacity for subluxation to progress, and only a few patients will eventually require surgery.

Erosion of the facet joints and osteoporosis are usually secondary mechanisms compounding the effects of ligamental laxity and disc disorder. The resultant effect can lead to neurological compression of either nerve root or spinal cord, presenting with brachiomyelopathy. This can be arrested but usually proceeds with gradual functional loss and disability.

9.6 **Clinical presentation**

Neck pain is a common feature in RA. It is usually associated with disc or facet joint disorder and with associated ligamental laxity and high nerve root compression (C2; C3). High nerve root compression can cause a headache (posterior occipital) associated with movement. Most patients respond to a combination of NSAIDs and DMARDs together with judicious use of external arthrodesis (soft or semi-rigid cervical collars). This may be limited, however, by skin abrasions and poor patient compliance.

Arm pain can be due to a number of reasons, ranging from limb joint disorder to nerve root compression. Patients with the latter typically present with paraesthesia and arm pain radiating in the relevant nerve root distribution. It can be difficult to separate peripheral nerve impingement from neuropathies and joint pains. This makes the diagnosis a significant challenge, requiring significant clinical experience and suspicion. A low threshold for imaging and neurophysiology helps in separating out the various causes.

Motor weakness and dysfunction can be equally difficult to separate out from the various causes for limb dysfunction. Modern imaging techniques have greatly changed the diagnosis of cord compression. The presence of a lower motor neurone sign (nerve root compression) may mask an upper neurone sign and lead to delayed diagnosis of spinal cord compression. Paraesethesia in the upper limbs should trigger early cervical spine MRI.

9.7 **Investigation**

Axial and sub-axial deformity can be monitored by plain AP and lateral X-rays during conservative therapy. Measurement of PADI will provide an estimate of cord compression. Post-operatively, X-rays are used to measure stabilization and calcification at the operative level and changes at the adjacent segments. CT scanning is not a useful diagnostic tool but can be used pre and post operatively to measure dimensions for screw placement and determine the position of the vertebral artery, particularly its course within the lateral mass of C2. Magnetic resonance imaging (MRI) allows accurate resolution of spinal cord and nerve root compression. Dynamic MRI can also be used to resolve the effect of poor stability, particularly in sub-axial disease.

9.8 Therapy

The progression of cervical spine problems in rheumatoid arthritis is usually slow, developing over months and years. Conservative management has an important role to play. The soft cervical collar, whilst biomechanically inefficient in stabilizing the spine, can promote natural fusion, thereby avoiding the use of internal fixation.

A collar can be used to prevent spinal movement whilst the patient is mobile in order to maintain the cervical spine in the correct position. Patients with severe neck instability will need a collar for constant support of the head or to reduce pain. With lesser degrees of instability, a collar could be used when patients are in a car or during prolonged activity when the neck could adopt extreme positions of flexion.

Custom made collars accommodate the deformities found in rheumatoid arthritis and may correct cervical spine subluxation in up to 50% of patients Problems with collars include patient acceptability, potential for development of pressure sores especially with more rigid collars, difficulties of applying and removing collars, and wear of the collar with use .

Surgical intervention has radically changed over the last decade with the introduction of lateral mass screw/polyaxial systems showing significant advantage over wire/fixed rod systems.

9.8.1 Wire fixation

Spinous process wires may fail due to decalcification and poor bone structure despite adequate bone grafting. Sub-laminar wires with rod systems have better results but rely on the presence of a generous spinal canal diameter and solid calcification in the lamina, neither of which are common in RA.

9.8.2 Screw fixation systems

The lateral mass maintains high levels of cortical calcification in the rheumatoid neck despite structural deformity. This provides good fixation if the fixation system can adapt to abnormal anatomy. The addition of poly-axial heads to the screws allows variable attachment to rods, and stabilizes the subluxation. The risks of damage to the vertebral artery and exiting nerve roots are low (5% injury to vertebral artery and less than 1% for nerve root injury). Pedicle screws are used as a 'salvage' procedure if the lateral mass proves inadequate; they require a lateral approach with wide muscle dissection.

9.8.3 Complications

Surgical complications are rare. Rates of infection, haematoma and haemorrhage are similar to other cervical spine operations with similar rates of neurological damage (1:500 tetraplegia). Delayed complications occur in fewer than 10%, often from loosening of screws and implants, because of a delay in bone fusion in RA. Patients classically experience 'clicking'. These symptoms should be investigated with dynamic flexion/extension X-rays. Polyaxial systems require CT scanning to detect fractures and slipped rods and screws. The routine use of bone grafts remains controversial because bone quality from the donor site may be poor quality.

9.8.4 Outcomes

The most effective aspects of segmental fixation in cervical spine surgery are control of neck pain and prevention of further neurological deterioration. More than 90% of patients with uncontrollable neck pain improve with surgical stabilization. Patients who are bed ridden by myelopathy have a high mortality without surgery (60% over 6 months); surgical intervention, whilst challenging for both the patient and the hospital team, has a significantly lower mortality (10–20% over 6 months) and the majority regain the capacity to feed themselves and many regain mobility.

9.8.5 Prognosis

Patients with RA are living longer with higher levels of independence due to a number of factors; changes in disease state, improved medical therapy, anaesthetic and surgical techniques. Short (C0 to C4/5) craniocervical (CC) fusion preserves neck movement, but may need to be extended subsequently to include the thoracic spine. By contrast, craniothoracic fusion (C0 to T2/3) is technically more successful, but has the limitation of complete loss of neck movement. Earlier C1/C2 fusion protects against basilar invagination and prevents the need for trans-oral surgery. An earlier small operation reduces the incidence of more extensive debilitating surgery.

9.9 Conclusion

The advances of medical and surgical treatment have revolutionised the outcome of rheumatoid arthritis patients. The early introduction of DMARDs and the use of TNF inhibitors have improved disease control. The resulting maintenance of bone density and strength has led to improvement in both conservative and surgical outcomes. General health has also improved and older patients can withstand complex cervical spine operations with lower overall mortality and shorter inpatient stays.

Further reading

Kauppi M, Hakala M. Prevalence of cervical spine subluxations and dislocations in a community-based rheumatoid arthritis population. *Scand J Rheumatol.* 1994; **23**(3): 133–6.

Kauppi M. Conservative treatment for rheumatoid cervical spine. *Lancet.* 1996; **347**(9016): 1695.

Menezes AH, van Gilder JC. Transoral-transpharyngeal approach to the anterior craniocervical junction. Ten-year experience with 72 patients. *J Neurosurg.* 1988; **69**(6): 895–903.

Neva MH, Häkkinen A, Mäkinen H, Hannonen P, Kauppi M, Sokka T. High prevalence of asymptomatic cervical spine subluxation in patients with rheumatoid arthritis waiting for orthopaedic surgery. *Ann Rheum Dis.* 2006; **65**(7): 884–8.

Chapter 10

Surgical management of rheumatoid arthritis: the upper limb

Ian McNab and Chris Little

Key points

- Pain from synovitis of the acromioclavicular joint localizes to the joint and responds to intra-articular steroid or arthroscopic excision of the lateral end of the clavicle
- Pain from gleno-humeral disease that does not improve with articular injections is best managed by humeral head replacement, but glenoid bone loss generally makes glenoid resurfacing inadvisable
- Rotator cuff impingement and tears that do not respond to injections and scapular control exercises are best treated by arthroscopic subacromial decompression and debridement
- Arthroplasty will usually reduce pain and improve function, particularly in the flail elbow, but carries increased surgical risks and a higher likelihood of loosening than other large joint replacements
- Nerve compression around the elbow is common, but often relatively asymptomatic
- Olecranon bursal excision surgery is usually avoided due to the low but significant risks of inadequate wound healing
- If hand function deteriorates and pain progresses or increases despite maximal medical therapy, surgical intervention is indicated.

10.1 The shoulder in rheumatoid arthritis

10.1.1 Acromio-clavicular joint

This is commonly affected by rheumatoid synovitis, often with radiographic changes, but because symptoms are similar to those of rotator cuff disease it is important to determine the source of pain. Box 10.1 shows the typical features of ACJ involvement.

Initial treatment is by intra-articular steroid. Since the orientation of the joint varies (lateral clavicle often over- or under-rides the acromion) a plain radiograph helps to indicate the best angle for the needle. Surgery should be considered if this fails; excision arthroplasty (arthroscopically removing the lateral centimetre of the clavicle) improves symptoms in 80% of patients.

10.1.2 Gleno-humeral joint

The radiographic pattern of disease may be "dry" (with loss of joint space, bony sclerosis and marked stiffness), "wet" (with marked synovitis, marginal humeral head erosions and central glenoid erosion) or "resorptive" (with marked bone loss, often with glenoid loss down to or beyond the coracoid process). Intra-articular steroid injections can give good transient relief. The degree of bone loss, particularly from the glenoid, often makes total shoulder replacement inadvisable, due to problems with securely fixing a glenoid component in place; hemi-arthroplasty is preferred, giving good pain control but limited improvement in function.

10.1.3 Rotator cuff

Impingement pain occurs at the deltoid insertion on arm elevation (Figure 10.2), but if pain is present at rest and at night, a rotator cuff tear is probably present (seen in up to 40%). Loss of movement due to pain or altered shoulder mechanics are seen if the tear is large (this will give rise to a lag sign, with the patient unable to maintain the position of the passively-placed arm, indicating a massive tear). Initial non-operative treatment is indicated with steroid injections into the subacromial bursa and physiotherapy to improve scapular positioning.

> ### Box 10.1 Typical features of ACJ involvement in RA
>
> - Pain well localized to the joint
> - Pain reproduced by high arc (>120 degrees – end of range) elevation movements (abducting the outstretched arm above the patients head) and by horizontal flexion (crossing the arm towards the opposite shoulder when elevated by 90 degrees; the 'scarf test')
> - Tenderness over ACJ.

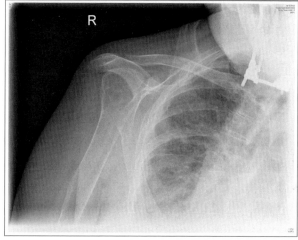

Figure 10.1 **X-ray of shoulder showing significant bone loss, particularly from the glenoid, making total shoulder replacement inadvisable in this case**

Rotator cuff repair is often technically difficult due to poor tissue quality, which results in a high rate of repeat tears. Arthroscopic surgery to decompress and debride the bursa often helps those patients who respond transiently to non-operative treatments (even those with full thickness cuff tears). Fistula formation from the arthroscopic port sites is more common than in non-rheumatoid patients.

10.2 The elbow in rheumatoid arthritis

10.2.1 Ulno-humeral and radio-carpal joints

Patients may develop diffuse pain around the elbow, stiffness, with loss of function, or instability due to bone erosion (Figure 10.3) and soft tissue attenuation ("flail elbow"). Radiographic changes often do not correlate with symptoms. Intra-articular steroid injections give transient relief. Patients with lateral pain and restricted forearm rotation benefit from radial head excision coupled with a synovectomy; however symptoms commonly recur. Components may be unlinked (surface replacement of the distal humerus and proximal ulna, with excision of the radial head), so that stability becomes dependent on soft tissue balance and reconstructions. Alternatively, linked components can be used (the humeral and ulnar components are connected, providing stability but potentially increasing mechanical loosening with

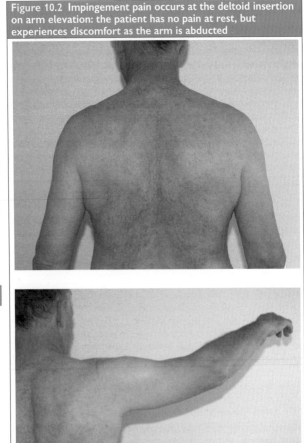

Figure 10.2 Impingement pain occurs at the deltoid insertion on arm elevation: the patient has no pain at rest, but experiences discomfort as the arm is abducted

time), particularly in flail elbows. "Sloppy hinge" implants allow a little varus/valgus tilt between linked components to minimise the risk of mechanical loosening.

In the absence of complications, pain control is usually good and motion improved by around 20 degrees of flexion/extension. The risk of infection or wound breakdown and nerve damage (ulnar nerve) is greater than with other commonly replaced large joints (hip/knee), and radiographic loosening is common but may be asymptomatic. The 5 year implant survival rate is 90%.

Figure 10.3 X-ray demonstrating elbow instability due to bone erosion

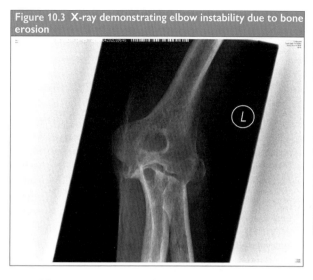

10.2.2 Ulnar nerve compression

Symptomatic ulnar nerve compression is uncommon in RA, although sub-clinical disease and neurophysiological changes are very common. Presentation is with intermittent tingling in the little and ring fingers (with or without objective sensory changes); intrinsic wasting (especially of the 1st dorsal interosseous muscle) or irritability of the ulnar nerve behind the medial epicondyle. Failure to improve with avoidance of local pressure and prolonged flexion is an indication for neurophysiological testing (to confirm nerve compression at the elbow) and a surgical review. Surgical decompression would not be recommended because it leaves the nerve in a "hostile" bed; anterior transposition is preferred.

10.2.3 Posterior interosseous nerve palsy

This is usually due to local compression by cysts from the elbow joint, compression by local fibrous bands or vasculitis. Presentation is with wrist drop and the inability to dorsiflex fingers at the MCP joint. It is important to exclude extensor tendon attrition rupture [due to tenosynovitis and distal radio ulnar joint (DRUJ) synovitis at the wrist; see Box 10.2 below] and extensor mechanism subluxation at the MCPJ as the cause of the dropped fingers. The treatment of choice is surgical exploration to decompress the nerve and remove any local synovitis.

Box 10.2 **Differential diagnosis of apparent finger extension lag**

- Posterior interosseous nerve palsy caused by elbow synovitis (examination reveals intact extensor tendons producing finger extension during maximal passive wrist flexion).
- Extensor tendon rupture (loss of both active finger extension and passive extension).
- EDC (extensor digitorum communis) tendon sagittal band rupture allowing subluxation of the extensor tendon into the valley between the metacarpal heads (if fingers are first placed in extension, allowing the extensor tendons to align centrally over the dorsum of the metacarpal heads, this position can be maintained actively, if fingers are first placed in flexion the subluxed extensor tendons cannot actively extend the MCP joints.
- Locked trigger finger (usually also has flexion of the PIP).
- Locked MCP joint (usually in OA with active and passive extension except for the last 40 degrees at MCP joint).
- Dupuytren's disease.

10.2.4 **Olecranon bursitis and rheumatoid nodules**

In patients with RA, the olecranon bursa is a common site of pressure and friction. Pressure avoidance with or without aspiration of the bursa is the initial treatment of choice. Surgical excision is possible, but carries the potential for delayed healing and sinus formation.

10.3 **The hand and wrist in rheumatoid arthritis**

Rapid improvements in medical treatment are starting to impact on the course and pattern of rheumatoid arthritis presenting to hand surgeons. However, RA continues to cause pain and impaired hand function, resulting in a need for reconstructive hand and wrist surgery.

10.3.1 **Patient assessment and planning surgery**

RA in the hand can affect multiple joints, but especially the wrist and distal radio ulnar joint (DRUJ), the metacarpo phalangeal (MCP) and proximal interphalangeal (PIP) joints of the fingers and the carpo metacarpal (CMC) and MCP joints of the thumb. In addition to the direct destruction of articulating joint surfaces, synovitis associated with RA causes attenuation and rupture of important joint stabilizing ligaments and tendons, which leads to progressive joint subluxation and dislocation, and to the development of several characteristic zigzag collapse deformities in the hand (Figure 10.4). Fibrosis and contracture of the intrinsic muscles of the hand also contributes to the development of finger deformities.

Initially, patients adapt their activities to accommodate their reduced hand function. However, if their hand function and pain continue to deteriorate despite maximal medical therapy, physiotherapy, occupational therapy, functional aids and resting splints, then they may require surgical intervention.

Patients with these complex and challenging hand and wrist problems require a highly integrated approach to their assessment (see Chapter 9, Box 9.2) and treatment. This is often best provided in a combined medical and surgical rheumatoid arthritis clinic. The extended multidisciplinary team includes rheumatologists, radiologists, nurses, physiotherapists, occupational therapists, hand surgeons and anaesthetists (see Box 10.3 below for a checklist prior to upper limb surgery).

The primary goals of surgical treatment are to help alleviate pain and to maintain or improve hand function. A secondary consequence of correcting deformities may also be an improved appearance of the hand.

Figure 10.4 Development of several characteristic zigzag collapse deformities in the hand in RA

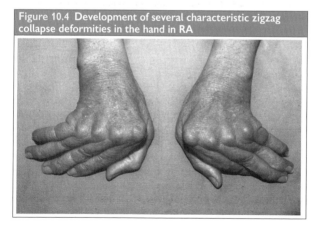

Box 10.3 Specific surgical assessment checklist prior to hand and forearm surgery (use in conjunction with general checklist in Box 9.2)

- Global upper limb examination: shoulder and elbow movements, positioning the hand in space for function (above the head, behind the back), adequate shoulder abduction and external rotation is required for axillary block anaesthesia and for placing the hand on the hand surgery operating table
- Test forearm rotation: supination and pronation requires free movement of both the proximal and distal radio ulnar joints (elbow and wrist)
- Assess DRUJ and extensor tendons
- Assess carpal tunnel and flexor tendons
- Wrist movement should be approximately 50:50 radiocarpal and mid carpal joint function
- Check thumb CMC and MCP and look for swan neck and boutonniere deformity
- Check fingers for MCP disease, ulnar drift or subluxation, abnormalities of PIPs and DIPs, and the presence of swan neck and boutonniere deformities
- Test the intrinsic muscles which flex the MCPs and extend the PIP joints and are placed under maximum tension when the MCP joints are passively extended and the PIP joints are passively flexed
- Intrinsic tightness test: compare PIP flexion with the MCP joint in extension versus flexion
- Assess skin and nails
- Neurovascular assessment.

The ultimate successful outcome of surgery for patients is determined not just by matching the correct patient to the correct procedure and meticulous attention to surgical detail and technique, but also by the multidisciplinary approach to postoperative rehabilitation. Extremely careful hand therapy is required following all of the procedures listed below.

10.3.2 Indications and timing of surgery

The indications for and the timing of surgery are discussed in the following sections relating to each anatomical region in the hand and wrist. However, these general principles must be carefully tailored to each individual patient's clinical presentation, general health, the current status of their rheumatoid arthritis, their optimal medications and the degree of disease control, the degree of existing physiotherapy and occupational therapy support, and their social and functional requirements and abilities (for home, work and hobbies).

In patients who require multiple surgical interventions, careful planning is required as to which order to perform the procedures in, and on which occasions. This initial plan may need to be adjusted as the programme of surgical treatment progresses. See chapter 9 for further discussion on timing of surgery.

If multiple level surgery is required in the upper limb itself, it is generally best to correct problems sequentially working from proximal towards more distal joints, or to address the most symptomatic or severely affected region first.

The concept of performing a "winner procedure" as the first operation is also important. These procedures need to have both predictable and good results that will hopefully ensure the patient's first experience of surgery is a positive one. Therefore, replacement arthroplasty of the shoulder or elbow, or arthrodesis (or arthroplasty) of the wrist is often undertaken first.

Occasionally, urgent surgery is required to prevent sudden further deterioration. For example, following rupture of the extensor tendons to the little finger, urgent excision of the ulnar head is required to prevent multiple extensor tendon ruptures.

10.3.3 DRUJ and extensor tendon surgery

Tenosynovitis (either flexor or extensor) that fails to respond to full medical treatment for 3–6 months (including steroid injection) may benefit from surgical tenosynovectomy, which may also reduce the rate of tendon rupture. Joint synovectomy may decrease symptoms but does not halt the progression of joint disease.

10.3.4 Caput ulnae syndrome

Caput ulnae syndrome is due to extensor tenosynovitis associated with DRUJ synovitis, leading to erosion and dorsal subluxation of the ulnar head through the dorsal joint capsule, plus extensor tendon rupture. Extensor digiti minimus and extensor digitorum communis (EDC) to the little finger usually rupture first causing an extensor lag to the little finger. The other EDC tendons may also go on to rupture sequentially from the ulnar side, creating a much more difficult reconstructive problem; rapid surgical intervention can prevent this. The surgical options are listed in Box 10.4.

Box 10.4 Surgical options for caput ulnae syndrome

- **Ulnar head excision plus soft tissue stabilization of the distal ulnar**: most commonly performed
- **Hemi-resection ulnar head plus soft tissue interposition/ stabilization**: in early disease
- **DRUJ arthrodesis plus pseudarthrosis proximal to the ulnar head**: can give unreliable results
- **Prosthetic ulnar head replacement (partial or total)**: established implants and techniques are available, but long-term results are not known
- **Extensor tenosynovectomy and tendon repairs, grafts or transfers, plus retinaculum transposition (deep to the tendons)**: usually combined with one of the above procedures
- **Rehabilitation following tendon reconstruction**: from 2 weeks post surgery gentle controlled range of motion exercises are commenced from a custom splint.

10.3.5 Carpal tunnel and flexor tendon problems

Flexor tenosynovitis associated with carpal tunnel syndrome may be the first presenting feature of RA. If it fails to respond to medical therapy to control synovitis or a steroid injection, it may require urgent carpal tunnel decompression with a flexor tenosynovectomy. Flexor tenosynovitis in the digits may cause triggering or reduce active range of motion, which can respond to medical management, failing which, a tenosynovectomy may be performed. Flexor pollicis longus (FPL) is the most common flexor tendon to rupture, due to palmar wrist synovitis and prominent bone spurs from the scaphoid and trapezium. If the thumb IP joint is stiff or ankylosed, then function may be maintained without intervention; otherwise, surgical reconstruction is indicated.

10.3.6 Wrist

Synovitis causes progressive attenuation and destruction of the intrinsic inter-carpal ligaments and the extrinsic intra-capsular ligaments of the wrist. The scapholunate ligament may rupture and the whole carpus slides down the articular surface of the radius into ulnar translation, palmar subluxation, and supination, with a secondary radial deviation of the metacarpals. The degree of surgical intervention required is matched to the level of the patient's pain and existing range of motion, the stage of the disease and to the pattern of joint destruction. Surgical options are listed in Box 10.5.

> **Box 10.5 Surgical options for wrist problems in RA**
>
> - Synovectomy (open or arthroscopic) may be useful in early disease
> - Extensor carpi radialis longus (ECRL) to extensor carpi ulnaris (ECU) transfer is useful if the wrist joint surfaces are still healthy
> - Radiolunate arthrodesis (or radioscapholunate arthrodesis) is indicated for isolated radiocarpal joint involvement, early ulnar translation of the carpus and preservation of >60 degrees arc of motion
> - Total wrist arthrodesis (using a dorsal wrist fusion plate, or inter-medullary metacarporadial pins) is indicated when both radiocarpal and mid carpal joints are involved
> - Total wrist arthroplasty techniques are evolving
> - Correction and stabilization of wrist subluxation and deformity.

10.3.7 Thumb

Common problems are summarized in Box 10.6.

> **Box 10.6 Common problems affecting the thumb**
>
> - **Boutonniere deformity:** MCP joint synovitis leads to extensor pollicis brevis (EPB) tendon rupture, weakness of proximal phalanx extension, and progressive "buttonholing" of the metacarpal head through the extensor apparatus. Extensor pollicis longus (EPL) subluxes anterior to the axis of MCP joint rotation, causing progressive flexion of the MCP joint and extension of the IP joint - a "Z collapse deformity"
>   - **Early flexible boutonniere deformity:** may be treated by transferring EPL on to the distal stump of EPB at the proximal phalanx base
>   - **Moderate late rigid boutonniere deformity (MCP flexion <45 degrees):** may be pain free and functional - requiring only occasional splintage
>   - **Painful severe late rigid boutonniere deformity (MCP flexion >45 degrees):** may be treated by MCP joint arthrodesis, plus lengthening of the EPL tendon, or IP joint arthrodesis, to reduce the disabling IP hyperextension
> - **Boutonniere deformity with associated CMC involvement:** requires correction of the metacarpal position by CMC excision arthroplasty, and an arthrodesis of the MCP joint
> - **Swan-neck deformity:** CMC joint synovitis attenuates the anterior oblique ligament causing dorsal subluxation of the metacarpal base, and a "thumb in the palm deformity". Associated progressive MCP hyperextension and EPL subluxation create the characteristic deformity.

Box 10.6 (Contd.)

- **Symptomatic disabling swan-neck deformity:** requires correction of the metacarpal position by CMC excision arthroplasty, and arthrodesis of the MCP joint
- **Thumb MCP joint ulnar collateral ligament insufficiency:** might be amenable to soft tissue reconstruction if the joint remains healthy, but often MCP joint arthrodesis is a more reliable procedure.

10.3.8 Metacarpophalangeal joints of the fingers

Common problems are summarized in Box 10.7.

Box 10.7 Common problems affecting finger MCP joints

- **MCP joint synovitis** causes attenuation of the joint capsule and collateral ligaments, and progressive ulnar drift and palmar subluxation of the base of the proximal phalanx
- **Ulnar drift** is multifactorial: there is a natural "push" towards MCP joint ulnar deviation caused by power gripping with the wrist in ulnar deviation; changes at the wrist cause the metacarpals to deform into radial deviation placing ulnar bias onto the EDC tendon's direction of pull; MCP joint synovitis also causes attenuation of the stabilizing sagittal bands and EDC tendon subluxation down the ulnar side of the metacarpal heads
- **Palmar subluxation** is driven by attenuation of the thin dorsal capsule, the powerful long flexor tendons to the fingers, and intrinsic muscle fibrosis and tightness
  - **Early MCP joint ulnar drift:** may be halted or corrected by the careful use of a resting night splint, and the modification of activities and walking aids etc. to minimize the ulnar deviation forces placed on the fingers
  - **Surgical intervention** to correct wrist deformities is also important when either preventing or correcting finger MCP joint ulnar deviation. **MCP joint synovectomy and soft tissue rebalancing (+/− crossed intrinsic transfer)** is occasionally useful in the presence of well preserved joint surfaces and synovitis resistant to medical intervention
  - **MCP joint silicon arthroplasty and soft tissue rebalancing (+/− crossed intrinsic transfer)** when performed carefully (often simultaneously on multiple fingers) can produce excellent results with good pain relief and correction of deformity, the maintenance of about 45+ degrees of flexion, and approximately 90% implant survival at five years. When the silicon spacer eventually fractures, if no symptoms or deformity develop, then no intervention is required.

10.3.9 Proximal interphalangeal joints of the fingers

Common problems are summarized in Box 10.8

Box 10.8 Common problems affecting finger PIP joints

- **PIP joint synovitis**, affecting predominantly the dorsal or palmar structures, in combination with intrinsic muscle contracture, results in the characteristic Z-shaped RA finger deformities
- **Boutonniere deformity:** this progressive deformity starts with the PIP joint synovitis causing attenuation of the central slip and weakness of PIP joint extension. The intrinsic muscles are employed increasingly in an attempt to extend the IP joints and the lateral bands sublux in a palmar direction, until they pass the axis of rotation and become flexors of the PIP joint. Intrinsic muscle action and contracture drives further PIP joint flexion and DIP joint extension
  - **Early mild flexible boutonniere deformity (PIPJ contracture <30 degrees):** may correct with a simple "Fowler's" release of the central third of the extensor tendon (performed at the junction of the proximal and middle thirds of the middle phalanx)
  - **Moderate flexible boutonniere deformity (PIPJ contracture >30 degrees):** if passively correctable with a healthy joint, the deformity may respond to a careful procedure to shorten the central slip with release and dorsal relocation and suturing of the lateral bands (+/- Fowler's release, for residual DIP joint hyperextension)
  - **Severe rigid boutonniere deformity (PIPJ contracture >60 degrees and DIPJ contracture >20 degrees):** if symptomatic, with such a poor range of PIP joint motion, the most reliable procedure is a PIP joint arthrodesis using K-wires and tension band (+/- Fowler's release, for residual DIP joint hyperextension)
- **Swan-neck deformity:** PIP joint synovitis causes attenuation of the palmar plate and the transverse retinacular ligament, allowing PIP joint hyperextension and dorsal subluxation of the lateral bands. Intrinsic muscle tightness and shortening of the extensor apparatus drive the finger further into MCP joint flexion, PIP joint hyperextension, and DIP joint flexion
  - **Early flexible swan-neck deformity:** during active flexion (possibly with some passive assistance) the finger may suddenly snap from hyperextension into flexion, often with some pain. Treatment options include extension block "silver ring" splint; stabilizing the palmar aspect of the PIP joint with a tenodesis using one of the flexor digitorium superficialis (FDS)

Box 10.8 (Contd.)

tendon slips; reconstructing the oblique retinacular ligament with the ulnar lateral band or a tendon graft; re-routing one lateral band through the flexor tendon sheath at the level of the PIP joint

• **Late rigid swan neck deformity:** if symptomatic, with PIP joint damage, the most reliable procedure is a PIP joint arthrodesis in a better position for function.

Further reading

Goldfarb CA, Dovan TT. Rheumatoid arthritis: silicone metacarpophalangeal joint arthroplasty indications, technique, and outcomes. *Hand Clin.* 2006; **22**(2): 177.

Simmen BR, Bogoch ER, Goldhahn J. Surgery Insight: orthopedic treatment options in rheumatoid arthritis. *Nat Clin Pract Rheumatol.* 2008; **4**(5): 266–73.

Soojian MG, Kwon YW. Elbow arthritis.Bull *NYU Hosp Jt Dis.* 2007; **65**(1): 61–71.

Thomas T, Noël E, Goupille P, Duquesnoy B, Combe B; GREP. The rheumatoid shoulder: current consensus on diagnosis and treatment. *Joint Bone Spine.* 2006; **73**(2): 139–43.

Trieb K. Treatment of the wrist in rheumatoid arthritis. *J Hand Surg [Am].* 2008; **33**(1): 113–23.

van de Sande MA, Brand R, Rozing PM.Indications, complications, and results of shoulder arthroplasty. *Scand J Rheumatol.* 2006; **35**(6): 426–34.

Chapter 11

Surgical approach to the lower limb in rheumatoid arthritis

Hemant Pandit, Bob Sharp and Roger Gundle

> ### Key points
>
> - Total hip and knee replacement (THR and TKR) are both very successful operations to relieve pain and improve function
> - Prostheses should usually be cemented because poor bone stock may not support cementless fixation
> - The risk of post operative sepsis is about twice as high in RA compared with osteoarthritis
> - The aim of forefoot management is to optimize comfort and function and to minimize the risk of skin breakdown or ulceration
> - Fusion of the first MTP joint and excision of the metatarsal heads for the patients suffering advanced forefoot disease leads to a very high level of patient satisfaction
> - Management options for patients with stiffened arthritic mid-foot joints include orthotics, shoe wear, analgesia and walking aids; surgery is rarely required
> - Many patients present with inflammation around the tendons particularly of the hind foot, which if untreated, may lead to rupture.

129

11.1 The hip and inflammatory joint disease

Hip involvement is common in RA. In a study of 103 patients followed for eight years from onset of an inflammatory arthropathy (97% of whom had rheumatoid factor), 20% had clinical evidence of hip joint involvement with 10% showing marked X-ray changes, 3% severe destruction and 1% protrusio acetabuli (Figure 11.1).

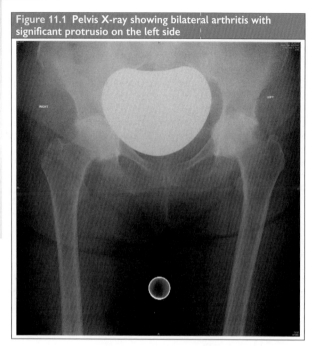

Figure 11.1 Pelvis X-ray showing bilateral arthritis with significant protrusio on the left side

11.1.1 Indications for surgical treatment of hip diseases

THR is most commonly used for end stage hip joint disease. Pain and immobility are the major indications for surgery. Multidisciplinary assessment is required before operation: the ability to use walking aids depends on upper limb function; feet should be examined for comfort in weight-bearing and as potential sources of sepsis. If foot surgery is required, it is best performed first because of a higher risk of post operative infection. There is commonly both hip and knee disease; hip surgery should be undertaken first because of reliable pain relief, functional gain and abolition of knee pain referred from the hip. Subsequent knee arthroplasty is also more satisfactory when the hip above is mobile; a rare exception might be when there is gross instability of the knee.

When there is severe symmetrical disease and particularly when there are significant bilateral fixed flexion deformities, simultaneous bilateral surgery should be considered to allow early mobilisation and prevent recurrence of deformity before the second side is treated. Similar considerations apply to bilateral knee disease with deformity.

11.1.2 Surgical options for the treatment of hip disease

Intra-articular injection of local anaesthetic and steroid is effective as well as being a useful diagnostic tool to localize pain. Owing to the deep location of the hip this should be undertaken in strict aseptic conditions and using image control by an experienced radiologist. Open surgical synovectomy of the hip is not a popular operation. Hip arthroscopy is becoming more widely practised and there are reports of symptomatic improvement after arthroscopic partial synovectomy in rheumatoid arthritis. Arthrodesis is not appropriate in patients with multiple joint disease and osteotomy is contraindicated because the disease is present throughout the joint. Hemiarthroplasty, commonly used to treat intracapsular fracture, is not recommended because it leaves behind acetabular articular cartilage which is pre-disposed to early wear.

THR is the preferred treatment option (Figure 11.2). On average patients are a decade younger than those with osteoarthritis presenting for THR. Hip replacement is associated with reduction in pain, improved sleep and walking ability and thus improved quality of life for these patients. The prosthesis should usually be cemented because poor bone stock with increased turnover may not support cementless fixation. Antibiotic impregnated bone cement is advisable given the increased risk of infection. Approximately 30% of patients coming for THR present with protrusio and this requires a bone graft to the medial wall of the acetabulum, usually an autograft from the proximal femur and neck. Complications of hip surgery are described in Table 11.1.

11.2 The knee in inflammatory joint disease

11.2.1 Synovectomy

Synovectomy is performed in order to relieve the patient's symptoms from the painful synovitis and also to prevent further damage to articular cartilage and adjacent bone. The use of effective disease modifying drugs and biologics has significantly reduced the need for surgical synovectomy.

Regenerated synovium after synovectomy is more fibrous with less inflammatory proliferative tissue. Indications and pre-requisites for patients for synovectomy are shown in Table 11.2.

Previously, synovectomy was performed with an open approach through a midline or parapatellar incision. However, this has largely been replaced by arthroscopic surgery using multiple portals, which allows faster recovery and with less morbidity.

Figure 11.2 Post-operative AP X-ray of left hip showing THR with bone grafting of the protrusion acetabuli

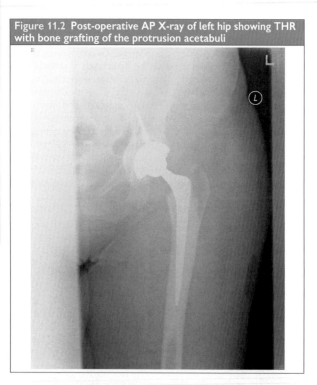

132

Table 11.1 Complications of hip surgery in RA	
Infection	Infection is the most feared complication (the risk is about twice as high as with osteoarthritis). This is due to immune dysfunction from the disease itself, often compounded by the effects of glucocorticoids, but probably not affected by use of DMARDs.
Thrombo-embolic disease	Appears to be is less common in rheumatoid arthritis compared with osteoarthritis.
Heterotopic ossification	A rare complication after THR in inflammatory joint disease.
Migration of the cemented acetabular cup	More common in rheumatoid arthritis than osteoarthritis suggesting that socket fixation is less secure. These data have led to interest in the use of cementless fixation of the acetabular component in THR in rheumatoid arthritis.

Table 11.2 Indications and pre-requisites for patients for synovectomy

- Persistent synovitis not responding to medical management over a period of three months.
- Preservation of useful range of movement.
- Absence of severe joint space (cartilage) loss.

11.2.2 Total Knee Replacement

TKR is a very successful operation to relieve pain in end stage knee disease in RA (Figures 11.3 and 11.4). Early diagnosis as well as adequate and prolonged disease control with effective DMARDs has resulted in a decline in the number of patients presenting for joint replacement with significant deformity. This has helped in earlier rehabilitation and reduced the need for the use of constrained implants.

Figure 11.3 Knee X-ray in a young woman showing severe loss of cartilage and secondary osteoarthritis due to RA

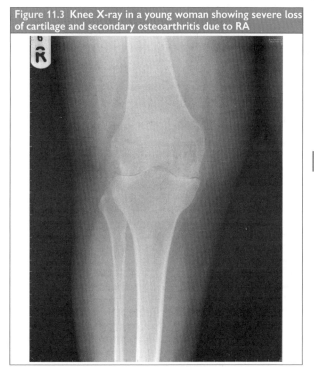

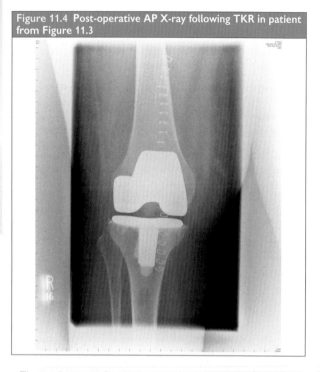

Figure 11.4 Post-operative AP X-ray following TKR in patient from Figure 11.3

134

The involvement of multiple joints does mean that patients with rheumatoid arthritis make fewer demands on their joints than do patients with other forms of chronic arthritis and therefore the life expectancy of prostheses may be longer. In patients undergoing TKR for inflammatory arthropathy, a higher infection rate and the development of late instability requiring revision surgery are the main concerns although with improved surgical techniques, the incidence of these is low. Some surgeons consider the presence of a plano-valgus foot as a forerunner of failure of a knee replacement in patients with inflammatory arthropathy.

Inflammatory arthritis is a good indication for resurfacing the patella while performing a TKR. This is because synovitis involving the extensor mechanism may contribute to peri-patellar pain in patients with rheumatoid arthritis. The prevalence of complications after patella resurfacing is lower in rheumatoid patients than in those with osteoarthritis because of lower functional demand. Partial (uni-compartmental) knee replacement is not indicated in patients with inflammatory arthropathy.

11.3 The foot and ankle in inflammatory joint disease

Improved medical management of rheumatoid arthritis has reduced the number of patients requiring foot surgery. However, many patients still require surgical input, although most can be managed with non-operative measures.

11.3.1 The hindfoot

The hind foot consists of the tibiotalar joint and the triple joints, namely the subtalar, calcaneocuboid and talonavicular joints. Hindfoot involvement is common in RA. Whilst non-operative measures should be pursued, some patients eventually require surgery. Joint and tendon disease leads to hindfoot valgus deformities (see Figure 11.5). Such mechanical derangements affect the rest of the foot and can lead to pressure sores and ulcers over bony prominences. Stress fractures may develop in the tibia and fibula as a result of the malposition of the hind foot beneath the leg.

Many patients with rheumatoid arthritis will spontaneously fuse their own triple joints, but not the ankle joint itself. In the hind foot, the aim of surgery is to enable the patient to place a plantigrade foot beneath the lower leg with the limb axis aligned. This usually involves a triple fusion. The associated poor skin and vascular supply favour a

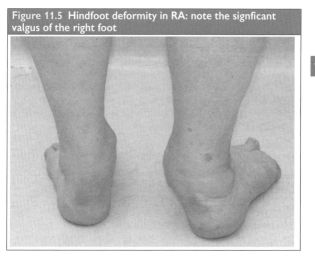

Figure 11.5 Hindfoot deformity in RA: note the signficant valgus of the right foot

medial approach in order to correct the hindfoot because this allows excision of redundant medial skin rather than tight closure of the lateral scar. Whilst arthroscopic techniques are being developed, triple fusion remains mostly an open surgical procedure. Plaster immobilization is required for 2–3 months.

The ankle is frequently affected in patients with rheumatoid arthritis. Early disease can be treated with injections of steroid or arthroscopic debridement. In more advanced disease, arthroscopic ankle fusion has a good outcome in terms of fusion rates and reduced wound complications. The alternative to fusion is an ankle replacement, with results similar to those seen in patients with OA. Arthroplasty has a higher initial complication rate including wound breakdown, neurovascular damage, implant malpositioning and failure and these can even require amputation. The immobility of the hindfoot with ankle fusion may adversely affect other involved joints in the lower limb and for this reason most surgeons would offer an ankle replacement to patients with multi-joint involvement.

Many patients with rheumatoid arthritis have problems at both the ankle and the triple hindfoot complex. A triple fusion would correct any deformity prior to a subsequent ankle replacement or an ankle fusion. Simultaneous ankle fusion and triple fusion is possible using an intramedullary nail through the calcaneum and talus into the tibia. This procedure is associated with higher risks but means that the patient only has one operation. The other option is to offer simultaneous hindfoot fusion and ankle replacement.

11.3.2 The mid-foot

Mid-foot joints are commonly involved in RA, but do not require surgery as frequently as the forefoot or hindfoot joints. Many patients spontaneously fuse their own mid-foot joints. Stiffened mid-feet can result in secondary effects on the forefoot because the loss of mobility of the mid-foot means the forefoot takes more abnormal loads. Management options for patients with stiffened arthritic mid-foot joints include X-ray guided injections, orthotics, modified shoes, analgesia and walking aids.

11.3.3 The forefoot

The classic deformities that occur in the forefoot of patients with rheumatoid arthritis (Table 11.3) result in discomfort, impair function and may lead to skin breakdown or ulceration.

Deformities can be managed with orthotics, pads and shoe modifications (see Chapter 7), but younger patients are reluctant to use orthopaedic shoes. For the lesser toes, surgical options include tendon release/lengthening and release of tight soft tissue structures around the joints. Shortening osteotomies allow reduction of the toes onto the

Table 11.3 Classical forefoot deformities in patients with RA	
Lesser toes: claw, mallet or hammer toes	These become fixed with deterioration; deformities plus skin changes of RA and abnormalities in the hindfoot leads to break-down of skin over the prominent knuckles and joints of the toes with ulceration and infection.
Great toe: usually MTP disease	Stifness, pain, malalignment; altered bio-mechanics lead to abnormal load across the foot with risks of ulceration or abnormal calluses due to pressure.
Associated rheumatoid nodules	Often found over bony prominences and predispose patients to pain, skin lesions and ulceration.

end of the metatarsals and recreate the normal functional apparatus of the toes, but they are not possible if there is destruction of the metatarsal heads, in which case bony resection is preferred. Conservative metatarsal surgery such as the Stainsby procedure involves removing some of the proximal phalanx to allow correction of the toe deformities while preserving the metatarsal heads. Joint preserving surgery should be used for the first ray if the MTP joint is preserved. Insertion of prosthetic joints or prosthetic hemiarthroplasties is not currently recommended. For more advanced cases, classical forefoot procedures are effective, such as fusion of the first MTP joint and excision of the metatarsal heads for the patients suffering advanced forefoot disease. However, whilst offering almost immediate relief of symptoms, over time, many patients develop callosities over the cut ends of the metatarsal heads more proximally in the foot. Further resections are not possible and reconstructive options have been eliminated.

11.3.4 **Soft tissue problems in the rheumatoid foot**
Many patients have rheumatoid nodules around their feet. These can occur in pressure areas over metatarsal or toe prominences which can cause discomfort and potentially ulcerate. These nodules can be removed with few risks of complications in the majority of patients; surgery should be offered if non-operative measures fail to control symptoms.

11.3.5 **Tenosynovitis**
Many patients present with inflammation around the tendons particularly of the hind foot, which, if untreated, may lead to rupture. Options include medical management, physiotherapy and splinting. Failing this, or in the presence of a rupture, debridement plus or minus reconstruction of the tendons should be performed. The Achilles tendon is not commonly affected in patients with RA and few ruptures seem to

occur. Tendonitis can be treated with non-operative measures such as physiotherapy and splinting. Experimental measures include shock-wave therapy, blood patches and dry needling of the tendon. Injections of steroid directly into the tendon should be avoided because of the risk of rupture.

11.3.6 Tibialis posterior tendon problems

The tibialis posterior tendon passes beneath the medial malleolus to support the medial side of the foot. This tendon holds the foot upright, holds the foot beneath the leg and maintains the arch of the foot. The tendon is frequently involved in patients with rheumatoid arthritis, leading to flat foot and collapse and a valgus hind foot. Surgical and medical management of a painful tendon should be proactive in order to prevent subsequent rupture.

Patients present with pain and tenderness around the medial malleolus and changing architecture of the foot. The patient's hind foot will be in valgus (see Figure 11.5) and does not correct into varus on tip toe and again when viewed from behind, the "too many toes" sign (see Figure 11.6) may be seen. Therapy involves reducing weight bearing through the foot, splinting, plaster of Paris and physiotherapy. Paratendonitis, i.e. inflammation around the tendon, can be treated with an injection of steroid under ultrasound guidance with the patient being put into plaster or a surgical splint following the injection to minimize the risk of rupture. Early disease not responding to conservative measures can be managed with arthroscopic or open

Figure 11.6 The "too many toes" sign in the left foot of a patient with valgus at the ankle due to RA

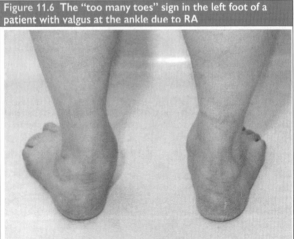

debridement. More advanced cases require tendon reconstruction with tendon transfers from elsewhere in the foot often in association with a medializing osteotomy to the back of the heel to alter the mechanics of the foot and to take some load off the medial structures.

11.3.7 Tendon ruptures in the foot

Tenosynovitis should be treated aggressively with medical therapy in the early stages in order to minimize the risk of rupture. The spring ligament lies on the under and medial surface of the foot and helps to maintain the arch. It can rupture spontaneously or in association with rupture or failure of the tibialis posterior tendon. Treatment is as for that described for tibialis posterior disease. Rupture of the anterior tendons should be treated surgically with immediate repair. Delayed repair is often difficult and involves tendon transfers.

Further reading

den Broeder AA, Creemers MC, Fransen J, de Jong E, de Rooij DJ, Wymenga A, de Waal-Malefijt M, van den Hoogen FH. Risk factors for surgical site infections and other complications in elective surgery in patients with rheumatoid arthritis with special attention for anti-tumor necrosis factor: a large retrospective study. *J Rheumatol.* 2007; **34**(4): 689–95.

Grondal L, Tengstrand B, Nordmark B, Wretenberg P, Stark A. The foot: still the most important reason for walking incapacity in rheumatoid arthritis: distribution of symptomatic joints in 1,000 RA patients. *Acta Orthop.* 2008; **79**(2): 257–61.

Kapetanovic MC, Lindqvist E, Saxne T, Eberhardt K. Orthopaedic surgery in rheumatoid arthritis patients over 20 years. Prevalence and predictive factors of large joint replacement. *Ann Rheum Dis.* 2008 Jan 4. [Epub ahead of print]

Molloy AP, Myerson MS. Surgery of the lesser toes in rheumatoid arthritis: metatarsal head resection. *Foot Ankle Clin.* 2007; **12**(3): 417–33.

Nguyen-Oghalai TU, Ottenbacher KJ, Caban M, Granger CV, Grecula M, Goodwin JS. The impact of rheumatoid arthritis on rehabilitation outcomes after lower extremity arthroplasty. *J Clin Rheumatol.* 2007; **13**(5): 247–50.

Trieb K, Schmid M, Stulnig T, Huber W, Wanivenhaus A. Long-term outcome of total knee replacement in patients with rheumatoid arthritis. *Joint Bone Spine.* 2008; **75**(2): 163–6.

Chapter 12

Future treatments in rheumatoid arthritis

Raashid Luqmani and Paul P Tak

Key points

- New treatments are required for the management of rheumatoid arthritis
- A greater understanding of disease mechanisms should allow the development of a more rational approach to therapy
- New strategies include combination biologic therapy, targeting of synovial fibroblasts, personalized therapy based on disease profiles, local gene therapy, and vaccination.

The last 15 years have seen a dramatic improvement in the management of rheumatoid arthritis with the introduction of the new biologic agents aimed at blocking TNF alpha, B cell function and co-stimulatory molecules such as CD28. However despite the radical improvement seen in some patients, the majority are still suffering from active disease. Most studies show that only 17% of patients have really effective therapy (equivalent to an ACR 70) although the majority of patients have more modest improvement. This suggests that there is a huge unmet need in the current management of rheumatoid arthritis. New therapeutic options would include combinations of biologic therapies, targeting of synovial fibroblasts, individualized therapies determined by personal profiles of biomarkers, local treatment for persistent joint disease or some kind of immunisation against pro-inflammatory molecules. We will look at some of these areas in a little more detail but they remain speculative as we are still exploring these ideas in their experimental phase. Furthermore some of the results from animal models may not be reflected in human practice. We will review some potential future developments as outlined in Box 12.1.

Box 12.1 Future developments in treatment of RA

- Combination biologic therapies
- Targeting of synovial fibroblasts
- Individualized, personalized therapy
- Local treatment
- Therapeutic vaccines

12.1 Combination biologic therapies

Blockade of pro-inflammatory cytokines like TNF or IL-6 in combination with for instance B cell depletion or inhibition of neoangiogenesis might be more effective than just single cytokine blockade. There is a concern that this might cause untoward effects in terms of interfering with the normal immune function. Another approach could be to address the cytokine cascade at a higher level such as the interference with IL-17 production by Th17 cells (see Chapter 2). IL-17 blockade may be effective in reducing joint inflammation and clinical trials in patients are currently underway.

12.2 Targeting of synovial fibroblasts

In addition to macrophages, T- and B-cells, fibroblast-like synoviocytes present in the joint directly contribute to joint destruction. These cells can enhance the production of matrix-degrading enzymes and induce excessive release of cytokines to boost the immune system. However, none of the currently available therapeutic strategies specifically interfere with these cells, which may explain persistent disease activity in a subset of the patients. Conceivably, new treatments could be developed which have a specific effect on activated synovial fibroblasts. Examples of such strategies include the development of extracellular signal-regulated kinase (ERK) inhibitors, and histone deacetylase (HDAC) inhibitors.

12.3 Individualized, personalized therapy

It is increasingly practical to perform gene array measures to look at the expression profile in an individual. With better technology this may be extended so that the whole genome can be studied providing a pattern of expression of genes. If these can be carefully identified then we can determine exactly which genes are being over expressed or under expressed, or patterns of genes, in an individual patient at any given time. The profiles may change with time and this might trigger a change in therapy and may help to explain why some therapies are only effective for certain lengths of time. This technology provides an opportunity to really look at individualized management.

12.4 Local treatment

The use of local treatment such as intra-articular steroids as an adjunct to systemic therapy has been very standard for many years but perhaps more innovative local treatment could be the introduction of gene therapy into joints. This is a practical alternative for patients who have achieved good control of their systemic arthritis and the majority of joints have improved whilst one or two joints might have persistent disease. There are considerable advantages to introducing treatment directly to the joint. If it is gene therapy then locally produced proteins can suppress the inflammation in the longer term and therefore the treatment may only be required on intermittent occasions to sustain the effect. It is currently possible to use harmless viruses such as the adeno-associated virus (AAV) as a vector to incorporate a human gene which is expressed over a long period of time by human cells at the site of inflammation. In animal models of arthritis, it is possible to inject AAV virus into joints and demonstrate its presence in synovial tissue. The most effective AAV for transduction of the inflamed synovium seems to be serotype 5. A potential gene of interest is interferon-beta which has anti-inflammatory effects. The other advantage of interferon-beta is that it can interfere with osteoclastogenesis, therefore inhibiting bone erosion. In some prototype experiments this has been done in a rat model of rheumatoid arthritis; interferon-beta was cloned into an AAV5 vector and was shown to transduce synovial tissue resulting in reduced inflammation and protection against joint destruction.

12.5 Therapeutic vaccines

Vaccination may become a reality for a number of diseases such as hypertension, obesity, osteoporosis and even cocaine or nicotine addiction. In rheumatoid arthritis the objective would be to use a vaccine to elicit an anti-cytokine response. One way is to combine TNF with a carrier protein and induce antibodies against TNF. This has been demonstrated in an animal model, both in preventing disease and also in treating established disease. In these animals, the vaccine has been shown to be as effective as the use of infliximab but provides more long lasting benefit. The other advantage of this vaccination is that it doesn't appear to cause complete TNF blockade and is therefore less likely to predispose to infection. An alternative to vaccinating with a whole molecule would be to use peptides which are the small amino acid components of larger cytokine molecules. For example, a peptide from IL-1 might be incorporated into a plasmid vector and vaccinated into patients and result in inhibiting the effects of IL-1. Similar efforts are being made for IL-17 and TGF (the latter for cancer patients).

12.6 **Conclusions**

A greater understanding of the immune system is driving a more rational approach to therapy and in the long term should have great benefits for patients. However we must avoid being overly optimistic. Specific targeting of what are essential housekeeping functions of the immune system might lead to predictable and sometimes unpredictable adverse outcomes which might make these approaches unsafe. Therefore continued vigilance and long term safety monitoring is going to be essential before the introduction of some of these agents into practice.

Further reading

Delavallée L, Le Buanec H, Bessis N, Assier E, Denys A, Bizzini B et al. Early and long-lasting protection from arthritis in tumour necrosis factor alpha (TNFalpha) transgenic mice vaccinated against TNFalpha. *Ann Rheum Dis.* 2008 Sep;**67**(9):1332–8.

Grabiec AM, Tak PP, Reedquist KA. Targeting histone deacetylase activity in rheumatoid arthritis and asthma as prototypes of inflammatory disease: should we keep our HATs on? *Arthritis Res Ther.* 2008;**10**(5):226.

Kramer I, Wibulswas A, Croft D, Genot E. Rheumatoid arthritis: targeting the proliferative fibroblasts. *Prog Cell Cycle Res.* 2003; **5**: 59–70.

Ospelt C, Neidhart M, Gay RE, Gay S.Synovial activation in rheumatoid arthritis. *Front Biosci.* 2004; **9**: 2323–34.

Vervoordeldonk MJ, Aalbers CJ, Tak PP. Advances in local targeted gene therapy for arthritis: towards clinical reality. *Future Rheumatol* 2008;**3**: 307–309

Index